THE CIRRHOSIS COOKBOOK

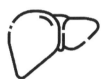

1000 Days of Delicious and Easy Recipes
To Improve Your Health with No Stress | Including
A 4-Stage Cirrhosis-Friendly Meal Plan

Charlie Pollys

Table of Contents

INTRODUCTION

The liver is the largest solid organ in the body and is responsible for several vital processes. The liver is an organ of the digestive system, having many functions including detoxification and protein synthesis as well as chemical generation to aid in food digestion. It is important to have a foundational understanding of the liver's structure and physiology in order to recognize the signs and symptoms of liver dysfunction.

When cirrhosis-caused organ damage prevents the digestive system from extracting the nutrients our bodies need from food in a timely manner, a diet designed specifically for this condition can ensure that our bodies get the nourishment they need without taxing the remaining healthy tissue. Patients with hepatic illnesses (especially hepatitis or cirrhosis) who don't get enough nutrition (especially protein) from their diets are at increased risk for consequences, including death, according to studies. In order to keep liver cirrhosis at bay, a healthy diet is essential. Scarring can worsen if it isn't treated, which can increase the chance of complications like cancer or organ bleeding.

If you have cirrhosis and are worried about the time and effort it would take to manage your diet, rest assured that there are a plethora of delicious and easy-to-follow recipes in this book.

Let's get started.

CHAPTER 1:
What is Cirrhosis

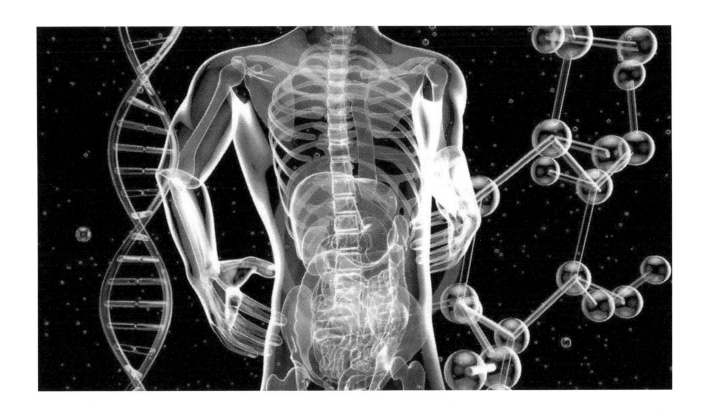

Cirrhosis of the liver

Liver cirrhosis is a progressive condition characterized by the gradual replacement of good liver tissue by scar tissue. The liver's capacity to metabolize nutrients, cleanse and process hormones and medicines, and so on, is adversely affected since the scar tissue literally blocks the flow of blood within the liver. A failing liver gradually becomes unable to perform its vital tasks.

Causes of liver cirrhosis

The most common causes of cirrhosis of the liver are fatty liver disease that is mostly associated with diabetes and obesity, excessive alcohol intake, and severe viral infections that affect your liver, such as Hepatitis B and C. Basically anything that has negative effects on your liver can lead to cirrhosis. There are some other causes of cirrhosis of the liver as well.

Autoimmune Diseases

Some people suffer from chronic illnesses that involve their own immune system launching an attack on their bile duct or liver cells. These include biliary cholangitis, autoimmune hepatitis, and multiple sclerosis, to mention a few.

Bile Duct Blockage

When bile is created in the liver, it is stored in the bile duct which then transports bile to your intestines where it helps digest fat. When the duct blocks, it is no longer able to carry out this function and, when the blockage is not addressed, it starts affecting your liver and can lead to cirrhosis.

Heart Failure Attacks

Repeated heart failure attacks lead to fluid backing up in the liver. This fluid can cause congestion that eventually leads to clogging of some of the ducts found in the liver.

Illnesses Associated With Abnormal Liver Function

An example of such an illness is hemochromatosis where more iron than what is needed is absorbed and supplied to the liver and other organs.

Glycogen Storage

Glycogen is created from carbs by your liver and is then converted to glucose which is then absorbed into your blood stream to provide energy. When your body is not able to convert glycogen into glucose, it leads to glycogen storage problems that could lead to cirrhosis if not addressed in a timely manner.

Common symptoms of cirrhosis of the liver

The symptoms are going to vary depending on what stage of cirrhosis you are in. At onset, there may be very little or no symptoms at all but then with the disease progression, you could start experiencing:

- Abnormally itchy skin
- Extreme sudden weight gain or weight loss
- Edema (fluid retention) manifesting as swollen legs, ankles and abdomen
- Traces of blood in your stool
- Extreme fatigue
- Dark brown or orange colored urine
- Loss of appetite
- Jaundice that manifests as the yellowing of the whites of your eyes or skin
- Light-colored stool (pointing to insufficient bilirubin)

- Unexplained bruising
- Sudden personality changes that include disorientation and confusion

One of the earliest signs of cirrhosis is edema which is basically retention of salt and fluid. It often manifests as a slightly swollen leg or ankle at first. With time, the fluid retention extends to your abdomen, a condition known as ascites. When identified early, your doctor will advise you to reduce your intake of salt and also prescribe diuretics. However, if you have a severe case of ascites, your doctor may need to drain the fluid. This is because if the fluid is not drained, it could lead to an infected abdomen, referred to as peritonitis.

If left unattended to and the fluid retention continues to the point it does not respond to any form of treatment, it could lead to the need for a liver transplant.

How to keep your liver healthy

It Starts With Food

As we have already seen, the liver is tasked with the metabolization of fats which, unlike proteins and carbs, are very difficult to digest. It's therefore prudent to avoid excessive consumption of fats to avoid overworking your liver which can lead to fatty liver disease, as is the case with people suffering from obesity.

Avoid Excessive Consumption Of Alcohol

Heavy alcohol consumption leads to cirrhosis of the liver over time. The process of your liver breaking down alcohol involves the production of free radicals and chemicals such as acetaldehyde. For serious damage to occur in your liver, it takes about a liter of wine, or its equivalent on a daily basis for 20 years in men. For women, it takes less than half of the amount to cause serious damage.

Take Caution When Taking Medication

Some medicinal combinations can be heavily taxing on your liver and it's always advisable that all medicines that you take are prescribed by a medical professional. Additionally, avoid mixing medication with natural remedies as this too can be overwhelming to your liver. It is especially important that you not mix alcohol with medicine as this can be too heavy on your liver, to the point of liver failure in extreme cases. It is important that you ask your doctor if it's okay to consume alcohol with the drugs you have been prescribed.

Avoid Aerosol/ Airborne Chemicals

When using gardening, housecleaning chemicals and paint, ensure that your environment is well ventilated and also put on a mask. Try as much as possible to reduce your inhalation of toxins as the liver is forced to process all toxins and this can cause liver problems, especially if you are exposed to toxic agents on a regular basis.

Practice Safe Sex

At the moment there is no vaccination for Hepatitis C. As such you should practice caution when it comes to sex, piercings and tattoos.

Get The Necessary Vaccinations

It is important that you get vaccinated especially if you are intending on travelling to a place where malaria or Hepatitis A and B may be a concern. Yellow Fever has been shown to lead to liver failure, and malaria grows and multiplies in your liver. Take the necessary precautions by taking the recommended vaccines and drugs.

Avoid Exposure To Foreign Blood And Germs

If you come in contact with another person's blood, you should get immediate medical attention. Also avoid sharing personal items such as needles and toothbrushes. Take care of yourself to avoid exposure to germs.

CHAPTER 2:
Foods To eat and foods to avoid

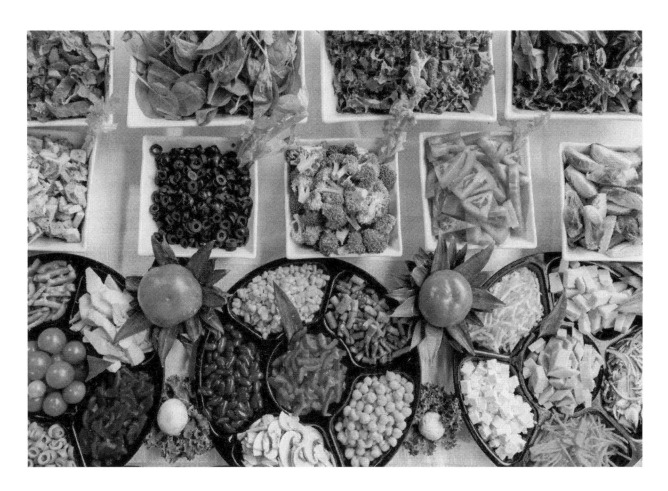

What to eat?

Broccoli

As per research, long haul utilization of broccoli forestalled fat development in the liver of mice. Cruciferous vegetables like spinach, cabbage, cauliflower are known to greatly benefit the liver.

Espresso

As indicated by a report distributed in the annals of hepatology, espresso contains certain aggravates that may help shield the body from non-alcoholic greasy liver ailment. Adding espresso to one's morning schedule might be a great option to prevent fat build-up in the liver.

Garlic

This common kitchen spice may help fix greasy liver illness. As indicated by advanced biomedical research, garlic seems to help reduce body weight and fat in individuals with greasy liver illness.

Green Tea

As indicated by the world journal of gastroenterology, tea, and particularly green tea, has elevated levels of cell reinforcements that help improve the muscle versus fat ratio and reduce fat in the blood.

Oatmeal

Whole grains like oatmeal contain slow-burning carbohydrates, that give your body energy for a longer duration and keep you feeling satiated. They are loaded with fiber content, which can help maintain your body weight. For a balanced and energizing breakfast, pair your oatmeal with a Tbsp. of nut butter like peanut or almond and sliced fruit.

Olive Oil

The presence of omega-3 unsaturated fats in olive oil help lower liver catalysts levels and control weight. So remember to use this oil for your fatty liver eating routine.

Pecans

Nuts rich in omega-3 unsaturated fats have extraordinary benefits for the liver. An investigation found that eating pecans improved liver capacity tests in individuals with non-alcoholic greasy liver malady.

Tofu

Tofu is known to reduce fat development in the liver. Besides, tofu is low in fat and high in protein that makes it a great choice for people with a fatty liver.

Sunflower Seeds

These crunchy delights are phenomenal wellsprings of Vitamin E, a cancer prevention agent which also shields the liver from harm. So remember to include these for your fatty liver eating regimen

Foods to avoid on a fatty liver diet

There are different types of foods that you should avoid or limit if you have a fatty liver. These foods contribute to weight gain and increase blood sugar.

Alcohol: Heavy and regular consumption of alcohol is a major cause of fatty liver disease as well as other liver diseases.

Salt: Consumption of too much salt can make your body hold excessive water. Sodium intake should be limited to less than 1,500 milligrams per day.

Sugar: Sugary foods such as candy, sodas, cookies, and fruit juices should be avoided. The amount of fat buildup in the liver is increased by high blood sugar.

Pasta, white bread and rice: White foods like pasta, white bread and white rice are highly processed, and tend to raise the blood sugar more rapidly compared to whole gains.

Saturated fats: Saturated fat includes red meat and butter. They should be avoided and instead replaced with healthy foods such as avocado, olive and cold-pressed nut oils.

Fried foods: Fried foods like chips, chicken wings and donuts are high in both fat and sugar, and are all-round bad for health.

The 4 stages of cirrhosis of the liver

Stage One: Inflammation

The first sign of liver disease is inflammation, causing it to be slightly enlarged and tender. Inflammation is usually a sign that your body is employing its natural defense tactics to fight an infection, heal injury or any foreign intrusion in order to restore health.

However, if inflammation keeps getting triggered the damage can exceed the benefit and can actually result in serious harm to your liver. The tricky thing about liver inflammation is that it does not cause any form of discomfort, unlike most other inflammations that will give you a sign that there is inflammation through redness, pain or elevated temperature. That is why it's very difficult to identify liver inflammation.

If, however, your doctor is able to identify inflammation in your liver during a routine checkup, it is possible to stop the problem that could be causing this before it progresses and causes serious and lasting damage. It is therefore important to schedule routine checkups.

Stage Two: Scarring Or Fibrosis

When inflammation is not identified, it leads to scarring that's formed every time the inflammation reduces only to come back again and again, considering how tender the liver is. This scarring when uncontrolled continues to the point that it replaces what used to be your healthy liver tissue. The bad thing about this is that scarred tissue cannot do the same work that your previously healthy liver tissue could. As more and more of fibrosis occurs, your liver tissue starts losing sensitivity and its functions start getting impaired as it has to work many times harder to get a simple job done.

If you are able to get an accurate diagnosis at this stage, your doctor will prescribe medication and a lifestyle change that will restore your liver to health in a relatively short duration.

Stage Three: Cirrhosis

Cirrhosis is the complete scarring of your entire liver, replacing the soft liver tissue with hard scar tissue. The liver will struggle and push to carry out its functions and, if not treated, will fail. In worst-case scenarios, will not be able to work at all.

This is where the symptoms start being visible. When you start experiencing the symptoms we outlined earlier, seek medical help immediately! Once you get the correct diagnosis, your doctor will focus on containing the disease so it does not progress. Once this has been achieved, the focus will shift to restoration which will be a deliberately slow process to ensure the damage is not exacerbated.

Stage Four: ESLD (End Stage Liver Disease)

At this stage, the liver is fully done in and there is very little chance of reversal as decompensation has occurred and the only option is a liver transplant. Decompensation usually includes an impairment of your kidney function, encephalopathy, lung problems, variceal bleeding and fluid retention in your abdomen that has to be physically drained. For this reason, such a patient is given priority in the liver transplant list.

So, how do you manage or treat liver cirrhosis?

Although there is no full cure for cirrhosis of the liver, there are treatments and management steps that help in delaying its progress and reducing its symptoms. This can reduce the complications that come with liver disease and also reduce the damage done to the liver cells.

Fluid retention in joints and the abdomen is first managed by following a very low sodium diet. For extreme cases of ascites, the doctor may have to drain the fluid from your stomach. Diuretics may also be prescribed to help reduce the fluid buildup.

If a patient's cirrhosis is a result of excessive alcohol consumption, then the first step is to refrain from any alcohol intake. This gives the liver a chance to take a break from the detoxification of blood brought about by alcohol consumption.

A healthy, low-sodium and balanced diet can be used to help improve the disorientation and confused mental conditions of patients. Sometimes laxatives may be prescribed to help absorb toxins, thus reducing the liver's job.

A lifestyle change that includes a healthy and natural low-sodium diet and daily physical activity is recommended to all patients as it helps the body heal itself by tapping into its primal self-healing ability.

For cirrhosis that was exacerbated by underlying medical conditions like autoimmune diseases, the doctor will start by addressing the underlying conditions and in some cases the damage can actually be reversed.

Patients with severe cirrhosis may need to get a liver transplant when all forms of treatment fail to respond and the damage to the liver continues to worsen.

In cases of autoimmune hepatitis, the doctor may prescribe drugs that suppress the immune system, such as azathioprine.

For hemochromatosis patients, treatment will involve removing blood in order to lower iron levels, thus preventing further liver damage. In cases of Wilson's disease, consisting of excess copper in the blood and liver, drugs will be administered to aid the removal of copper from the body through urine.

Do not use non-steroidal anti-inflammatory medications, including naproxen and ibuprofen. Patients with cirrhosis of the liver can further damage their livers and kidneys with such drugs.

Patients with Hepatitis C may need individualized treatment. The reason for this is that not all patients are in a position to receive antiviral treatment as it could lead to further liver damage in some cases. A doctor specializing in liver disease will carry out a series of tests to determine the best course of treatment.

Vaccinating patients with cirrhosis against Hepatitis A and B infections. This helps prevent further damage to the liver.

CHAPTER 3:
Breakfast Recipes

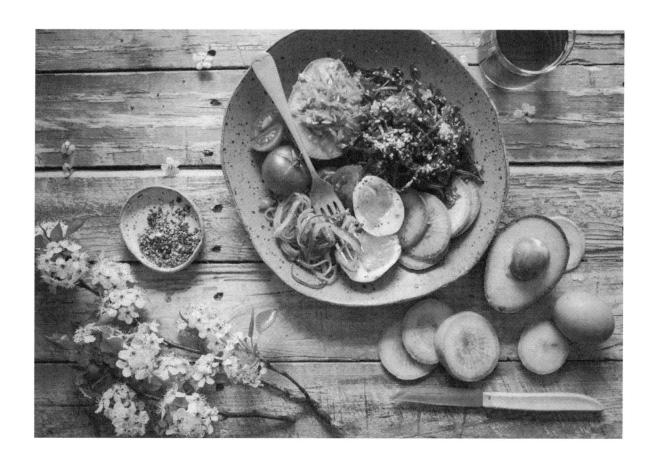

1. Spiced French toast

Prep time: 15 mins
Cooking time: 10 mins
Servings: 4
Ingredients:

- 4 eggs
- ½ cup homemade rice milk (or unsweetened store-bought) or almond milk
- ¼ cup freshly squeezed orange juice
- 1 tsp. ground cinnamon
- ½ tsp. ground ginger
- A pinch of ground cloves
- 1 Tbsp. unsalted butter, divided
- 8 slices white bread

Directions:

1. Whisk eggs, rice milk, orange juice, cinnamon, ginger, and cloves until well blended in a large bowl.
2. Melt half the butter in a large skillet. It should be on medium-high heat only.
3. Dredge four of the bread slices in the egg mixture until well soaked, and place them in the skillet.
4. Cook the toast until golden brown on both sides, turning once, about 6 minutes total.
5. Repeat with the remaining butter and bread.
6. Serve 2 pieces of hot French toast to each person.

Nutritional Facts: Calories 236; Total fat 11g; Saturated fat 4g; Cholesterol 220mg; Sodium 84mg; Carbs 27g; Fiber 1g; Phosphorus 119mg; Potassium 158mg; Proteins 11g.

2. Breakfast tacos

Prep time: 10 mins
Cooking time: 10 mins
Servings: 4
Ingredients:

- 1 tsp. olive oil
- ½ sweet onion, chopped
- ½ red bell pepper, chopped
- ½ tsp. minced garlic
- 4 eggs, beaten
- ½ tsp. ground cumin
- A pinch of red pepper flakes
- 4 tortillas
- ¼ cup tomato salsa

Directions:

1. Heat the oil in a large skillet, on medium heat only.
2. Add the onion, bell pepper, and garlic, and sauté until softened, about 5 minutes.
3. Add the eggs, cumin, and red pepper flakes, and scramble the eggs with the vegetables until cooked through and fluffy.
4. Spoon one-fourth of the egg mixture into the center of each tortilla, and top each with 1 Tbsp. of salsa.
5. Serve immediately.

Nutritional Facts: Calories 211; Total fat 7g; Saturated fat 2g; Cholesterol 211mg; Sodium 346mg; Carbs 17g; Fiber 1g; Phosphorus 120mg; Potassium 141mg; Proteins 9g.

3. Mexican scrambled eggs in tortilla

Prep time: 5 mins
Cooking time: 2 mins
Servings: 2
Ingredients:

- 2 medium corn tortillas
- 4 egg whites
- 1 tsp. of cumin
- 3 tsp. of green chilies, diced
- ½ tsp. of hot pepper sauce
- 2 Tbsp. of salsa
- ½ tsp. salt

Directions:

1. Spray some cooking spray on a medium skillet and heat for a few seconds.
2. Whisk the eggs with the green chilies, hot sauce, and cumin
3. Add the eggs into the pan, and whisk with a spatula to scramble. Add the salt.
4. Cook until fluffy and done (1-2 minutes) over low heat.
5. Open the tortillas and spread 1 Tbsp. of salsa on each.
6. Distribute the egg mixture onto the tortillas and wrap gently to make a burrito.
7. Serve warm.

Nutritional Facts: Calories: 44.1, Carbs 2.23g, Proteins 7.69g, Sodium 854mg, Potassium 189mg, Phosphorus 22mg, Fiber 0.5g, Fat 0.39g.

4. Avocado spread

Prep time: 10 mins
Cooking time: 0 mins
Servings: 4
Ingredients:

- 2 avocados, peeled, pitted and roughly chopped
- 1 Tbsp. sun-dried tomatoes, chopped
- 2 Tbsp. lemon juice
- 3 Tbsp. cherry tomatoes, chopped
- ¼ cup red onion, chopped
- 1 tsp. oregano, dried
- 2 Tbsp. parsley, chopped
- 4 kalamata olives, pitted and chopped
- A pinch of salt and black pepper

Directions:

1. Put the avocados in a bowl and mash with a fork.
2. Add the rest of the ingredients, stir to combine and serve as a morning spread.

Nutritional Facts: Calories 110, Fat 10g, Fiber 3.8g, Carbs 5.7g, Proteins 1.2g

5. Breakfast smoothie

Prep time: 15 mins
Cooking time: 0 mins
Servings: 2
Ingredients:

- Frozen blueberries – 1 cup
- Pineapple chunks – ½ cup
- English cucumber – ½ cup
- Apple – ½
- Water – ½ cup

Directions:

1. Put the pineapple, blueberries, cucumber, apple, and water in a blender and blend until thick and smooth.
2. Pour into 2 glasses and serve.

Nutritional Facts: Calories 87, Fat 12g, Carbs 22g, Phosphorus 28mg, Potassium 192mg, Sodium 3mg, Proteins 0.7g.

6. Carrot Omelette

Prep time: 10 mins
Cooking time: 5 mins
Servings: 4
Ingredients:

- 2 eggs
- ¼ tsp salt
- ¼ tsp black pepper
- 1 Tbsp. olive oil
- ¼ cup cheese
- ¼ tsp basil
- 1 cup carrot

Directions:

1. In a bowl, combine all ingredients together and mix well.
2. In a skillet, heat olive oil and pour the egg mixture.
3. Cook for 1-2 minutes per side.
4. When ready, remove omelette from the skillet and serve.

Nutritional Facts: Calories 320, Carbs 50g, Fat 11g, Proteins 10g.

7. Summer veggie omelette

Prep time: 5 mins
Cooking time: 5 mins
Servings: 2
Ingredients:

- 4 large egg whites
- ¼ cup of sweet corn, frozen
- ⅓ cup of zucchini, grated
- 2 green onions, sliced
- 1 Tbsp. of cream cheese
- Kosher pepper

Directions:

1. Grease a medium pan with some cooking spray and add the onions, corn and grated zucchini.
2. Sauté for a couple of minutes until softened.
3. Beat the eggs together with the water, cream cheese, and pepper in a bowl.
4. Add the eggs into the veggie mixture in the pan, and let cook while moving the edges from inside to outside with a spatula, to allow raw egg to cook through the edges.
5. Turn the omelet with the aid of a dish (placed over the pan and flipped upside down and then back to the pan).
6. Let sit for another 1-2 minutes.
7. Fold in half and serve.

Nutritional Facts: Calories 90, Carbs 15.97g, Proteins 8.07g, Sodium 227mg, Potassium 244.24mg, Phosphorus 45.32mg, Fiber 0.88g, Fat 2.44g.

8. Superfood liver cleansing soup

Prep time: 10 mins
Cooking time: 20 mins
Servings: 4
Ingredients:

- 1/4 cup water
- 2 cloves garlic, minced
- 1/2 of a red onion, diced
- 1 Tbsp. fresh ginger, peeled and minced
- 1 cup chopped tomatoes
- 1 small head of broccoli, florets
- 3 medium carrots, diced
- 3 celery stalks, diced
- 6 cups water
- 1/4 tsp. cinnamon
- 1 tsp. turmeric
- 1/8 tsp. cayenne pepper
- Freshly ground black pepper
- Juice of 1 lemon
- 1 cup purple cabbage, chopped
- 2 cups kale, torn into pieces

Directions:

1. Bring a large pot of water to a gentle boil over medium heat. Add garlic and onion and cook for about 2 minutes, stirring occasionally.
2. Stir in carrots, broccoli, tomatoes, fresh ginger, and celery and cook for another 3 minutes. Stir in cayenne, turmeric, cinnamon, and black pepper.
3. Add half cup of water to the pot and bring to a gentle boil; lower heat and simmer until the veggies get tender, for about 15 minutes.
4. Stir in kale, cabbage, and fresh lemon juice during the last 2 minutes of cooking. Serve hot or warm.

Nutritional Facts: 283.6 calories, 11.5g fat, 31g carbs, 10.9g proteins.

9. Sweet pancakes

Prep time: 10 mins
Cooking time: 5 mins
Servings: 5
Ingredients:

- All-purpose flour – 1 cup
- Granulated sugar – 1 Tbsp.
- Baking powder – 2 tsp.
- Egg whites – 2
- Almond milk - 1 cup
- Olive oil - 2 Tbsp.
- Maple extract – 1 Tbsp.

Directions:

1. Combine the flour, sugar and baking powder in a bowl.
2. Make a well in the center and place to one side.
3. Mix the egg whites, milk, oil, and maple extract in another bowl.
4. Add the egg mixture to the well and gently mix until a batter is formed.
5. Heat skillet over medium heat.
6. Cook 2 minutes on each side or until the pancake is golden (only add 1/5 of the batter to the pan).
7. Repeat with the remaining batter and serve.

Nutritional Facts: Calories 178, Fat 6g, Potassium 126mg, Sodium 297mg, Proteins 6g.

10. Mushroom-egg casserole

Prep time: 10 mins
Cooking time: 30 mins
Servings: 4
Ingredients:

- ½ cup mushrooms, chopped
- ½ yellow onion, diced
- 4 eggs, beaten
- 1 Tbsp. coconut flakes
- ½ tsp. chili pepper
- 1 oz. cheddar cheese, shredded
- 1 tsp. canola oil

Directions:

1. Pour canola oil in the skillet and preheat oven.
2. Add mushrooms and onion and roast for 5-8 minutes or until the vegetables are light brown.
3. Transfer the cooked vegetables in the casserole mold.
4. Add coconut flakes, chili pepper, and cheddar cheese.
5. Then add eggs and stir well.
6. Bake the casserole for 15 minutes at 360 F.

Nutritional Facts: Calories 152, Fat 11.1g, Fiber 0.7g, Carbs 3g, Proteins 10.4g.

11. Brown rice salad

Prep time: 10 mins
Cooking time: 0 mins
Servings: 4
Ingredients:

- 9 oz. brown rice, cooked
- 7 cups baby arugula
- 15 oz. canned garbanzo beans, drained and rinsed
- 4 oz. feta cheese, crumbled
- ¾ cup basil, chopped
- A pinch of salt and black pepper
- 2 Tbsp. lemon juice
- ¼ tsp. lemon zest, grated
- ¼ cup olive oil

Directions:

1. In a salad bowl, combine the brown rice with the arugula, the beans and the rest of the ingredients.
2. Toss and serve cold for breakfast.

Nutritional Facts: Calories 473, Fat 22g, Fiber 7g, Carbs 53g, Proteins 13g.

12. Cauliflower hash brown breakfast bowl

Prep time: 10 mins
Cooking time: 10 mins
Servings: 2
Ingredients:

- 1 Tbsp. lemon juice
- 1 egg
- 1 avocado
- 1 tsp. garlic powder
- 2 Tbsp. extra virgin olive oil
- 2 oz. mushrooms, sliced
- ½ green onion, chopped
- ¼ cup salsa
- ¾ cup cauliflower rice
- ½ small handful baby spinach
- Salt and black pepper, to taste

Directions:

1. Mash together avocado, lemon juice, garlic powder, salt and black pepper in a small bowl.
2. Whisk eggs, salt and black pepper in a bowl and keep aside.
3. Heat half of olive oil over medium heat in a skillet and add mushrooms.
4. Sauté for about 3 minutes and season with garlic powder, salt, and pepper.
5. Sauté for about 2 minutes and dish out in a bowl.
6. Add rest of the olive oil and add cauliflower, garlic powder, salt and pepper.
7. Sauté for about 5 minutes and dish out.
8. Return the mushrooms to the skillet and add green onions and baby spinach.
9. Sauté for about 30 seconds and add whisked eggs.
10. Sauté for about 1 minute and scoop on the sautéed cauliflower hash browns.
11. Top with salsa and mashed avocado and serve

Nutritional Facts: Calories 400, Carbs 15.8g, Fats 36.7g, Proteins 8g, Sodium 288mg, Sugar 4.2g.

13. Bacon, vegetable and parmesan combo

Prep time: 10 mins
Cooking time: 30 mins
Servings: 2
Ingredients:

- 2 slices of bacon, thick-cut
- ½ Tbsp. mayonnaise
- ½ of medium green bell pepper, deseeded and chopped
- 1 scallion, chopped
- ¼ cup grated parmesan cheese
- 1 Tbsp. olive oil

Directions:

1. Switch on the oven, then set its temperature to 375°f and let it preheat.
2. Meanwhile, take a baking dish, grease it with oil, and add slices of bacon in it.
3. Spread mayonnaise on top of the bacon, then top with bell peppers and scallions, sprinkle with parmesan cheese and bake for about 25 minutes until cooked thoroughly.
4. When done, take out the baking dish and serve immediately.
5. For meal prepping, wrap bacon in a plastic sheet and refrigerate for up to 2 days.
6. When ready to eat, reheat bacon in the microwave and then serve.

Nutritional Facts: Calories 197, Fat 13.8g, Carbs 4.7g, Proteins 14.3g, Sugar 1.9g, Sodium 662mg.

14. Herbed spinach frittata

Prep time: 10 mins
Cooking time: 20 mins
Servings: 4
Ingredients:

- 5 eggs, beaten
- 1 cup fresh spinach
- 2 oz. parmesan, grated
- 1/3 cup cherry tomatoes
- ½ tsp. dried oregano
- 1 tsp. dried thyme
- 1 tsp. olive oii

Directions:

1. Chop the spinach into the tiny pieces and or use a blender.
2. Then combine together chopped spinach with eggs, dried oregano and thyme.
3. Add parmesan and stir the frittata mixture with the help of the fork.
4. Brush the springform pan with olive oil and pour the egg mixture inside.
5. Cut the cherry tomatoes into the halves and place them over the egg mixture.
6. Preheat the oven to 360F.
7. Bake the frittata for 20 minutes or until it is solid.
8. Chill the cooked breakfast till the room temperature and slice into the servings

Nutritional Facts: Calories 140, Fat 9.8g, Fiber 0.5g, Carbs 2.1g, Proteins 11.9g.

15. Breakfast tostadas

Prep time: 10 mins
Cooking time: 20 mins
Servings: 4
Ingredients:

- ½ white onion, diced
- 1 tomato, chopped
- 1 cucumber, chopped
- 1 Tbsp. fresh cilantro, chopped
- ½ jalapeno pepper, chopped
- 1 Tbsp. lime juice
- 6 corn tortillas
- 1 Tbsp. canola oil
- 2 oz. cheddar cheese, shredded
- ½ cup white beans, canned, drained
- 6 eggs
- ½ tsp. butter
- ½ tsp. sea salt

Directions:

1. Make pico de galo: in a salad bowl, combine together diced white onion, tomato, cucumber, fresh cilantro, and jalapeno pepper.
2. Then add lime juice and a ½ Tbsp. of canola oil. Mix up the mixture well. Pico de galo is ready.
3. After this, preheat the oven to 390 F.
4. Line a tray with baking paper.
5. Arrange the corn tortillas on the baking paper and brush with remaining canola oil from both sides.
6. Bake the tortillas for 10 minutes or until they start to be crunchy.
7. Chill the cooked crunchy tortillas well.
8. Meanwhile, toss the butter in the skillet.
9. Crack the eggs in the melted butter and sprinkle them with sea salt.
10. Fry the eggs until the egg whites become white (cooked), approximately for 3-5 minutes over medium heat.
11. After this, mash the beans until you get puree texture.
12. Spread the bean puree on the corn tortillas.
13. Add fried eggs.
14. Then top the eggs with pico de galo and shredded cheddar cheese.

Nutritional Facts: Calories 246, Fat 11.1g, Fiber 4.7g, Carbs 24.5g, Proteins 13.7g.

16. Pasta with Indian lentils

Prep time: 10 mins
Cooking time: 35 mins
Servings: 4
Ingredients:

- ¼-½ cup fresh cilantro (chopped)
- 3 cups water
- 2 small dry red peppers (whole)
- 1 tsp. turmeric
- 1 tsp. ground cumin
- 2-3 cloves garlic (minced)
- 1 can diced tomatoes (w/juice)
- 1 large onion (chopped)
- ½ cup dry lentils (rinsed)
- ½ cup orzo or tiny pasta

Directions:

1. Combine all ingredients in the skillet, except for the cilantro, then boil on medium-high heat.
2. Ensure to cover and slightly reduce heat to medium-low and simmer until pasta is tender, for about 35 minutes.
3. Afterwards, take out the chili peppers then add cilantro and top it with low-fat sour cream.

Nutritional Facts: Calories 175; Carbs 40g; Proteins 3g; Fat 2g; Phosphorus 139mg; Potassium 513mg; Sodium 61mg.

17. Banana pancakes

Prep time: 10 mins
Cooking time: 10 mins
Servings: 4
Ingredients:

- 1 cup whole wheat flour
- ¼ tsp baking soda
- ¼ tsp baking powder
- 1 cup mashed banana
- 2 eggs
- 1 cup milk

Directions:

1. In a bowl, combine all ingredients together and mix well.
2. Heat some olive oil in a skillet.
3. Pour ¼ of the batter and cook each pancake for 1-2 minutes per side.
4. When ready, remove from heat and serve.

Nutritional Facts: Calories 210, Carbs 7g, Fat 14g, Proteins 15g.

CHAPTER 4:
Lunch Recipes

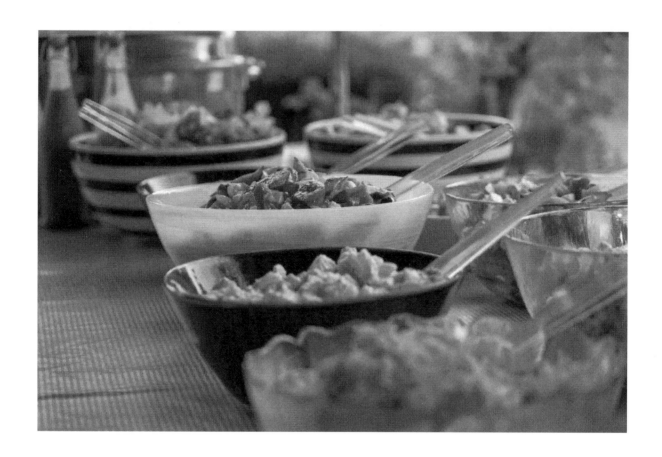

18. Roasted red endive with caper butter

Prep time: 10 mins
Cooking time: 25 mins
Servings: 4
Ingredients:

- 10 – 12 red endives
- 2 tsp. extra virgin olive oil
- 2–5 anchovy fillets, packed in oil
- 1 small lemon, juiced
- 3 Tbsp. capers, drained
- 5 Tbsp. cold butter, cut into cubes
- 1 Tbsp. fresh parsley, chopped
- Salt and pepper as needed

Directions:

1. Preheat the oven to 425 degrees F.
2. Toss endives with olive oil, salt, and pepper, and spread out on to a baking sheet, cut side down. Bake for about 20-25 minutes or until caramelized.
3. While they're roasting, add the anchovies to a large pan over medium heat and use a fork to mash them until broken up.
4. Add lemon juice and mix well, then add the capers.
5. Lower the heat and slowly stir in the butter and parsley.
6. Drizzle butter over roasted endives, season as necessary and garnish with more fresh parsley.

Nutritional Facts: Calories 109, Fat 8.6g, Proteins 1.5 g, Carbs 4.9 g, Fiber 4 g.

19. Zucchini pepper chips

Prep time: 10 mins
Cooking time: 15 mins
Servings: 4
Ingredients:

- 1 2/3 cups vegetable oil
- 1 tsp. garlic powder
- 1 tsp. onion powder
- 1/2 tsp. black pepper
- 3 Tbsp. crushed red pepper flakes
- 2 zucchinis, thinly sliced

Directions:

1. Mix oil with all the spices in a bowl.
2. Add zucchini slices and mix well.
3. Transfer the mixture to a Ziplock bag and seal it.
4. Refrigerate for 10 minutes.
5. Spread the zucchini slices on a greased baking sheet.
6. Bake for 15 minutes and serve hot.

Nutritional Facts: Calories 172, Total fat 11.1 g, Saturated fat 5.8 g, Cholesterol 610 mg, Sodium 749 mg, Total carbs 19.9 g, Fiber 0.2 g, Sugar 0.2 g, Proteins 13.5 g.

20. Apple chips

Prep time: 5 mins
Cooking time: 45 mins
Servings: 4
Ingredients:

- 2 golden apples, cored and thinly sliced
- 1 1/2 tsps. white sugar
- 1/2 tsp. ground cinnamon

Directions:

1. Set your oven to 225 degrees F.
2. Place apple slices on a baking sheet.
3. Sprinkle sugar and cinnamon over the apple slices.
4. Bake for 45 minutes.
5. Serve hot.

Nutritional Facts: Calories 127, Total fat 3.5 g, Saturated fat 0.5 g, Cholesterol 162 mg, Sodium 142 mg, Total carbs 33.6g, Fiber 0.4 g, Sugar 0.5 g, Proteins 4.5 g.

21. Creamy salmon soup

Prep time: 10 mins
Cooking time: 15 mins
Servings: 4
Ingredients:

- 2 Tbsp. olive oil
- 1 red onion, chopped
- Salt and white pepper to taste
- 3 gold potatoes, peeled and cubed
- 2 carrots, chopped
- 4 cups fish stock
- 4 oz. salmon fillets, boneless and cubed
- ½ cup heavy cream
- 1 Tbsp. dill, chopped

Directions:

1. Heat up a pan with the oil over medium heat, then add onion and sauté for 5 minutes.
2. Add the rest of the ingredients expect the cream, salmon and the dill, bring to a simmer and cook for 5-6 minutes more.
3. Add the salmon, cream and the dill, simmer for 5 minutes more, divide into bowls and serve.

Nutritional Facts: Calories 214, Fat 16.3g, Fiber 1.5g, Carbs 6.4g, Proteins 11.8g.

22. Tasty lime cilantro cauliflower rice

Prep time: 10 mins
Cooking time: 10 mins
Servings: 4
Ingredients:

- 1 head cauliflower, rinsed
- 1 Tbsp. extra-virgin olive oil
- 2 garlic cloves, minced
- 2 scallions, chopped
- ½ tsp. sea salt
- Pinch of pepper
- 4 Tbsp. fresh lime juice
- 1/4 cup chopped fresh cilantro

Directions:

1. Chop cauliflower into florets and transfer to a food processor; pulse into rice texture.
2. Heat a large skillet over medium heat and add olive oil; sauté garlic and scallions for about 4 minutes or until fragrant and tender.
3. Increase heat to medium high and stir in cauliflower rice; cook, covered, for about 6 minutes or until cauliflower is crispy on the outside and soft inside.
4. Season with salt and pepper and transfer to a bowl. Toss with freshly squeezed lime juice and cilantro and serve right away.

Nutritional Facts: Calories 300, Fat 17g, Saturated fat 4g, Cholesterol 16mg, Sodium 59mg, Carbs 34g, Fiber 2g, Proteins 7g.

23. Garlicky peas and clams on veggie spiral

Prep time: 10 mins
Cooking time: 15 mins
Servings: 4
Ingredients:

- 2 Tbsp. chopped fresh basil
- ½ cup pre-shredded parmesan cheese
- 1 cup frozen green peas
- ¼ tsp. crushed red pepper
- ¼ cup dry white wine
- 1 cup organic vegetable broth
- 3 cans chopped clams, clams and juice separated
- 1 ½ tsp. bottled minced garlic
- 2 Tbsp. olive oil
- 6 cups zucchini spiral

Directions:

1. Bring a pot of water to a boil and blanch zucchini for 4 minutes on high fire. Drain and let stand for a couple of minutes to continue cooking.
2. On medium high flame, place a large nonstick saucepan and heat oil. Add the garlic and sauté for a minute. Pour in wine, broth and clam juice.
3. Once liquid is boiling, reduce to a simmer and add pepper. Continue cooking and stirring for 5 minutes.
4. Add peas and clams, cook until heated through or around two minutes.
5. Toss in the zucchini, mix well. Cook until heated through.
6. Add basil and cheese, toss to mix well then remove from the stove.
7. Transfer equally to four serving bowls and enjoy.

Nutritional Facts: Calories 210; Carbs 24g; Proteins 8.5g; Fat 9.2g.

24. Chickpea fried eggplant salad

Prep time: 10 mins
Cooking time: 10 mins
Servings: 4
Ingredients:

- 1 cup chopped dill
- 1 cup chopped parsley
- 1 cup cooked or canned chickpeas, drained
- 1 large eggplant, thinly sliced (no more than 1/4 inch in thickness)
- 1 small red onion, sliced in 1/2 moons
- 1/2 English cucumber, diced
- 3 roma tomatoes, diced
- 3 Tbsp. za'atar spice, divided
- Oil for frying, preferably extra virgin olive oil
- Juice of 1 large lime
- 1/3 cup extra virgin olive oil
- 1–2 garlic cloves, minced
- Salt & pepper to taste

Directions:

1. On a baking sheet, spread out sliced eggplant and season with salt generously. Let it sit for 30 minutes. Then pat dry with a paper towel.
2. Place a small pot on medium high flame and fill halfway with oil. Heat oil for 5 minutes. Fry eggplant in batches until golden brown, around 3 minutes per side. Place cooked eggplants on a paper towel-lined plate.
3. Once the eggplants have cooled, assemble the eggplant on a serving dish. Sprinkle with 1 Tbsp. of za'atar.
4. Mix dill, parsley, red onions, chickpeas, cucumbers, and tomatoes in a large salad bowl. Sprinkle remaining za'atar and gently toss to mix.
5. Whisk well the vinaigrette ingredients in a small bowl. Drizzle 2 Tbsp. of the dressing over the fried eggplant. Add remaining dressing over the chickpea salad and mix.
6. Add the chickpea salad to the serving dish with the fried eggplant.
7. Serve and enjoy.

Nutritional Facts: Calories 642; Proteins 16.6g; Carbs 25.9g; Fat 44g.

25. Artichoke feta penne

Prep time: 10 mins
Cooking time: 30 mins
Servings: 4
Ingredients:

- 8 oz. Penne pasta
- 2 Tbsp. olive oil
- 1 shallot, chopped
- 4 garlic cloves, chopped
- 1 jar artichoke hearts, drained and chopped
- 1 cup diced tomatoes
- ¼ cup white wine
- ½ cup vegetable stock
- Salt and pepper to taste
- 4 oz. feta cheese, crumbled

Directions:

1. Heat the oil in a skillet and stir in the shallot and garlic. Cook for 2 minutes until softened.
2. Add the artichoke hearts, tomatoes, wine and stock, as well as salt and pepper.
3. Cook on low heat for about 15 minutes.
4. In the meantime, cook the penne in a large pot of water until al dente, not more than 8 minutes.
5. Drain the pasta well and mix it with the artichoke sauce.
6. Serve the penne with crumbled feta cheese.

Nutritional Facts: Calories 325, Fat 14.4g, Proteins 11.1g, Carbs 35.8g.

26. Creamy artichoke lasagna

Prep time: 10 mins
Cooking time: 60 mins
Servings: 4
Ingredients:

- 1 cup shredded mozzarella cheese
- 2 cups light cream
- ¼ cup all-purpose flour
- 1 cup vegetable broth
- ¾ tsp. salt
- 1 egg
- 1 cup snipped fresh basil
- 1 cup finely shredded parmesan cheese
- 1 15-oz. carton ricotta cheese
- 4 cloves garlic, minced
- ½ cup pine nuts
- 3 Tbsp. olive oil
- 9 dried lasagna noodles, cooked, rinsed in cold water and drained
- 15 fresh baby artichokes
- ¼ cup lemon juice
- 3 cups water

Directions:

1. Mix together lemon juice and water and put aside. Slice off the artichoke base and remove yellowed outer leaves then cut into quarters. Immediately soak the sliced artichokes in the prepared liquid and drain after a minute.
2. Over medium flame, place a big saucepan with 2 Tbsp. oil and fry half of garlic, pine nuts and artichokes. Stir frequently and cook until artichokes are soft, for around ten minutes. Turn off the fire and transfer the mixture to a big bowl and quickly stir in salt, egg, ½ cup of basil, ½ cup of parmesan cheese and ricotta cheese. Mix thoroughly.
3. In a small bowl, mix flour and broth. In the same pan, add 1 Tbsp. oil and fry the remaining garlic for half a minute. Add light cream and flour mixture. Stir constantly and cook until thickened. Remove from fire and stir in ½ cup of basil.
4. In a separate bowl, mix ½ cup parmesan and mozzarella cheese.
5. Assemble the lasagna by layering the following in a greased rectangular glass dish: lasagna, 1/3 of artichoke mixture, 1/3 of sauce, sprinkle with the dried cheeses and repeat layering procedure until all ingredients are used up.

6. Bake the lasagna in a pre-heated oven at 350 degrees F for 40 minutes. Remove lasagna from the oven and let it stand for 15 minutes before serving.

Nutritional Facts: Calories 425; Carbs 41.4g; Proteins 21.3g; Fat 19.8g.

27. Cod and mushrooms mix

Prep time: 10 mins
Cooking time: 20 mins
Servings: 4
Ingredients:

- 2 cod fillets, boneless
- 4 Tbsp. olive oil
- 4 oz. mushrooms, sliced
- Sea salt and black pepper to taste
- 12 cherry tomatoes, halved
- 8 oz. lettuce leaves, torn
- 1 avocado, pitted, peeled and cubed
- 1 red chili pepper, chopped
- 1 Tbsp. cilantro, chopped
- 2 Tbsp. balsamic vinegar
- 1 oz. feta cheese, crumbled

Directions:

1. Put the fish in a roasting pan, brush it with 2 Tbsps. oil, sprinkle salt and pepper all over and broil under medium-high heat for 15 minutes. Meanwhile, heat up a pan with the rest of the oil over medium heat, add the mushrooms, stir and sauté for 5 minutes.
2. Add the rest of the ingredients, toss, cook for 5 minutes more and divide between plates.
3. Top with the fish and serve right away.

Nutritional Facts: Calories 257, Fat 10g, Fiber 3.1g, Carbs 24.3g, Proteins 19.4g.

28. Oat risotto with mushrooms, kale, and chicken

Prep time: 10 mins
Cooking time: 30 mins
Servings: 4
Ingredients:

- 4 cups reduced-sodium chicken broth
- 1 Tbsp. extra-virgin olive oil
- 1 small onion, finely chopped
- 1 lb. sliced mushrooms
- 1 lb. boneless, skinless chicken thighs, cut into bite-size pieces
- 1¼ cups quick-cooking steel-cut oats
- 1 (10-oz.) package frozen chopped kale (about 4 cups)
- ½ cup grated parmesan cheese (optional)
- Freshly ground black pepper (optional)

Directions:

1. In a medium saucepan, bring the broth to a simmer over medium-low heat.
2. Warm the olive oil in a large, non-stick skillet over medium-high heat. Sauté the onion and mushrooms until the onion is translucent, for about 5 minutes. Push the vegetables to the side, and add the chicken. Let it sit untouched until it browns, about 2 minutes.
3. Add the oats. Cook for 1 minute, stirring constantly. Add ½ cup of the hot broth, and stir until it is completely absorbed. Continue stirring in broth, ½ cup at a time, until it is absorbed and the oats and chicken are cooked, for about 10 minutes. If you run out of broth, switch to hot water.
4. Stir in the frozen kale, and cook until it's warm. Top with parmesan and black pepper, if you like.
5. Flavor boost: garnish with minced parsley and red pepper flakes. You can also substitute ½ cup dry white wine for ½ cup of the chicken broth.
6. Ingredient tip: all varieties of oats have similar amounts of fiber, vitamins, and minerals. The main difference is in how quickly they're digested, with the steel-cut and old-fashioned/rolled oats breaking down more slowly, which is helpful for blood sugar control. The quick-cooking steel-cut oats used in this risotto are simply cut into smaller pieces, enabling you to make this dish in under 30 minutes.

Nutritional Facts: Calories 470, Fat 16g, Saturated fat 4g, Cholesterol 118mg, Sodium 389mg, Carbs 44g, Fiber 9g, Proteins 40g.

29. Turkey with leeks and radishes

Prep time: 10 mins
Cooking time: 6 hours
Servings: 4
Ingredients:

- 1-lb. turkey breast, skinless, boneless and cubed
- 1 leek, sliced
- 1 cup radishes, sliced
- 1 red onion, chopped
- 1 Tbsp. olive oil
- A pinch of salt and black pepper
- 1 cup chicken stock
- ½ tsp. sweet paprika
- ½ tsp. coriander, ground
- 1 Tbsp. cilantro, chopped

Directions:

1. In your slow cooker, combine the turkey with the leek, radishes, onion and the other ingredients. Toss them well put the lid on and cook on high for 6 hours.
2. Divide everything between plates and serve.

Nutritional Facts: Calories 226, Fat 9g, Fiber 1g, Carbs 6g, Proteins 12g.

30. Creamy green pea pasta

Prep time: 10 mins
Cooking time: 15 mins
Servings: 4
Ingredients:

- Packaged spaghetti
- Frozen peas - 1 cup
- Mascarpone or ricotta cheese - 1 cup
- Grated Parmesan - 1 cup
- Garlic, 4-5 cloves
- Fresh herbs for the sauce and seasoning

Directions:

1. Pour a few cups of water in a deep pot and bring to a boil with a pinch of salt.
2. Add the spaghetti and cook for 8 minutes then drain well.
3. For the sauce, combine the remaining ingredients in a blender and pulse until smooth. Then add to a medium frying pan and cook on low heat until it simmers.
4. Mix the cooked the spaghetti with the sauce, top with herbs of your choice and serve the pasta fresh.

Nutritional Facts: Calories 294, Fat 20.1g, Proteins 6.4g, Carbs 25.9g.

31. Smoked salmon and watercress salad

Prep time: 10 mins
Cooking time: 0 mins
Servings: 4
Ingredients:

- 2 bunches watercress
- 1 lb. smoked salmon, skinless, boneless and flaked
- 2 tsp. mustard
- ¼ cup lemon juice
- ½ cup Greek yogurt
- Salt and black pepper to taste
- 1 big cucumber, sliced
- 2 Tbsp. chives, chopped

Directions:

1. In a salad bowl, combine the salmon with the watercress and the rest of the ingredients and toss and serve right away.

Nutritional Facts: Calories 244,   Fat 16.7g,   Fiber 4.5g,   Carbs 22.5g,   Proteins 15.6g.

32. Blackened fish tacos with slaw

Prep time: 10 mins
Cooking time: 10 mins
Servings: 4
Ingredients:

- 1 Tbsp. olive oil
- 1 tsp. chili powder
- 2 tilapia fillets
- 1 tsp. paprika
- 4 low carb tortillas
- Slaw: ½ cup red cabbage, shredded
- 1 Tbsp. lemon juice
- 1 tsp. apple cider vinegar
- 1 Tbsp. olive oil
- Salt and black pepper to taste

Directions:

2. Season the tilapia with chili powder and paprika. Heat olive oil in a skillet over medium heat.
3. Add tilapia and cook until blackened, about 3 minutes per side. Cut into strips. Divide the tilapia between the tortillas. It's ready to serve.

Nutritional Facts: Calories 268, Fat 20g, Carbs 5g, Proteins 18g.

33. Easy mozzarella & pesto chicken casserole

Prep time: 10 mins
Cooking time: 30 mins
Servings: 4
Ingredients:

- ¼ - cup pesto
- 8 - oz. cream cheese, softened
- ¼ - ½ - cup heavy cream
- 8 - oz. mozzarella cubed
- 2 - lb. cooked cubed chicken breasts
- 8 - oz. mozzarella shredded

Directions:

1. Preheat stove to 400 degrees F.
2. Blend together the pesto, cream cheese, heavy cream and cubed mozzarella. Now add the chicken to this mix.
3. Transfer to a greased baking tray, sprinkle the shredded mozzarella on top and bake for 25-30 minutes.

Nutritional Facts: Calories 404, Fat 23g, Carbs 8g, Proteins 31g.

34. Beef bourguignon

Prep time: 10 mins
Cooking time: 1 hour 30 mins
Servings: 4
Ingredients:

- 3 Tbsp. olive oil
- 2 lb. beef roast, cubed
- 1 Tbsp. all-purpose flour
- 3 sweet onions, chopped
- 2 carrots, sliced
- 4 garlic cloves, minced
- 1 chili pepper, sliced
- 1 lb. button mushrooms
- 1 ½ cups beef stock
- ½ cup dark beer
- 2 bay leaves
- 1 thyme sprig
- 1 rosemary sprig
- Salt and pepper to taste

Directions:

1. Sprinkle the beef with flour.
2. Heat oil in a deep, heavy pot and add the beef.
3. Cook on all sides for 5 minutes or until browned.
4. Add the garlic, onions, carrots and chili, and cook for 5 more minutes.
5. Add the mushrooms, stock, beer, bay leaves, thyme, rosemary, salt and pepper.
6. Cover the pot and cook on low heat for 1 ½ hours.
7. Serve the stew warm and fresh.

Nutritional Facts: Calories 306, Fat 12.6g, Proteins 37.6g, Carbs 9.0g.

35. Feta, eggplant and sausage penne

Prep time: 10 mins
Cooking time: 10 mins
Servings: 4
Ingredients:

- ¼ cup chopped fresh parsley
- ½ cup crumbled feta cheese
- 6 cups hot cooked penne
- 1 14.5 oz can diced tomatoes
- ¼ tsp. ground black pepper
- 1 tsp. dried oregano
- 2 Tbsp. tomato paste
- 4 garlic cloves, minced
- ½ lb. bulk pork breakfast sausage
- 4 ½ cups cubed and peeled eggplant

Directions:

1. On medium high flame, place a nonstick frying pan and cook garlic, sausage and eggplant for about 7 minutes or until eggplants are soft and sausage are lightly browned.
2. Stir in diced tomatoes, black pepper, oregano and tomato paste. Cover and simmer for five minutes while occasionally stirring.
3. Remove pan from fire, stir in pasta and mix well.
4. Transfer to a serving dish, garnish with parsley and cheese before serving.

Nutritional Facts: Calories 376; Carbs 50.8g; Proteins 17.8g; Fat 11.6g.

36. Garlic mushroom chicken

Prep time: 10 mins
Cooking time: 10 mins
Servings: 4
Ingredients:

- 3 garlic cloves, minced
- 1 onion, chopped
- 2 cups mushrooms, sliced
- 1 Tbsp. olive oil
- ½ cup chicken stock
- 2 whole chicken breasts
- ¼ tsp. pepper
- ½ tsp. salt

Directions:

1. Season the chicken with pepper and salt. Heat oil in a pan on medium heat, then put the seasoned chicken in the pan and cook for 5-6 minutes on each side. Remove and place on a plate.
2. Add the onion and mushrooms to the pan and sauté until tender, about 2-3 minutes. Add garlic and sauté for another minute. Add the stock and bring to a boil. Stir well and cook for 1-2 minutes. Pour over the chicken and serve.

Nutritional Facts: Calories 331, Fat 14.5g, Proteins 43.9g, Carbs 4.6g, Sodium 420 mg.

37. Healthy chicken orzo

Prep time: 10 mins
Cooking time: 15 mins
Servings: 4
Ingredients:

- 1 cup whole wheat orzo
- 1 lb. Chicken breasts, sliced
- ½ tsp. red pepper flakes
- ½ cup feta cheese, crumbled
- ½ tsp. oregano
- 1 Tbsp. fresh parsley, chopped
- 1 Tbsp. fresh basil, chopped
- ¼ cup pine nuts
- 1 cup spinach, chopped
- ¼ cup white wine
- ½ cup olives, sliced
- 1 cup cherry tomatoes, cut in half
- ½ Tbsp. garlic, minced
- 2 Tbsp. olive oil
- ½ tsp. pepper
- ½ tsp. salt

Directions:

1. Heat 1 Tbsp. of olive oil in a pan over medium heat. Season chicken with pepper and salt and cook in the pan for 5-7 minutes on each side. Remove from pan and set aside.
2. Add water in a small saucepan and bring to a boil. Add orzo in the boiling water and cook according to the packet directions.
3. Heat the remaining olive oil in a pan on medium heat, then put garlic in the pan and sauté for a minute. Stir in white wine and tomatoes and cook on high flame for 3 minutes.
4. Add cooked orzo, spices, spinach, pine nuts, and olives and stir until well combined. Add chicken on top of the orzo and sprinkle with feta cheese. Serve and enjoy.

Nutritional Facts: Calories 518, Fat 27.7g, Proteins 40.6g, Carbs 26.2g, Sodium 121mg.

38. Lemony lamb and potatoes

Prep time: 10 mins
Cooking time: 2 hours 10 mins
Servings: 3
Ingredients:

- 2 lb. lamb meat, cubed
- 2 Tbsp. olive oil
- 2 springs rosemary, chopped
- 2 Tbsp. parsley, chopped
- 1 Tbsp. lemon rind, grated
- 3 garlic cloves, minced
- 2 Tbsp. lemon juice
- 2 lb. baby potatoes, scrubbed and halved
- 1 cup veggie stock

Directions:

1. In a roasting pan, combine the meat with the oil and the rest of the ingredients, then place it in a baking tray and bake at 400 degrees F for 2 hours and 10 minutes.
2. Divide the mix between plates and serve.

Nutritional Facts: Calories 302, Fat 15.2g, Fiber 10.6g, Carbs 23.3g, Proteins 15.2g.

39. Oven vegetables with salmon fillet

Prep time: 10 mins
Cooking time: 30 mins
Servings: 4
Ingredients:

- 250 g salmon fillet
- 1 medium zucchini
- 1 red pepper
- 300 g cherry tomatoes
- 150 g mushrooms
- 100 g of low-fat feta
- 1 Tbsp. olive oil
- Salt and pepper

Directions:

1. Preheat the oven to 180 degrees.
2. Rub the salmon fillet with salt and pepper.
3. Wash the zucchini and cut into large pieces. Wash the peppers, remove the core and cut into strips. Wash the cherry tomatoes and cut in half. Clean the mushrooms then cut off the hard stem ends and quarter. Put the vegetables and mushrooms in a bowl, drizzle with the olive oil, season with salt and pepper, and mix well.
4. Drain the feta and cut into cubes.
5. Spread the vegetables in a baking dish, sprinkle with the feta cubes and add the salmon fillet on top.
6. Cook on the middle rack for 30-35 minutes.
7. Take out of the oven, let cool down a little and serve.

Nutritional Facts: Calories 300, Fat 17g, Saturated fat 4g, Cholesterol 16mg, Sodium 59mg, Carbs 34g, Fiber 2g, Proteins 7g.

40. Pastitsio

Prep time: 10 mins
Cooking time: 30 mins
Servings: 4
Ingredients:

- 2 Tbsp. chopped fresh flat leaf parsley
- ¾ cup shredded mozzarella cheese
- 1 3-oz. package of fat-free cream cheese
- ½ cup 1/3 less fat cream cheese
- 1 can 14.5-oz. of diced tomatoes, drained
- 2 cups fat-free milk
- 1 Tbsp. all-purpose flour
- ¾ tsp. kosher salt
- 5 garlic cloves, minced
- 1 ½ cups chopped onion
- 1 Tbsp. olive oil
- 1 lb. ground sirloin
- Cooking spray
- 8 oz. penne, cooked and drained

Directions:

1. On medium high flame, place a big nonstick saucepan and sauté beef for five minutes. Keep on stirring to break up the pieces of ground meat. Once cooked, remove from the pan and drain the fat.
2. Using the same pan, heat some oil and fry onions until soft, around four minutes, while occasionally stirring.
3. Add garlic and continue cooking for another minute while stirring constantly.
4. Stir in the beef and flour, and cook for another minute. Stir constantly.
5. Add the fat free cream cheese, less fat cream cheese, tomatoes and milk. Cook until the mixture is smooth. Toss in the pasta and mix well.
6. Transfer the pasta into a greased rectangular glass dish and top with mozzarella. Cook in a preheated broiler for four minutes. Remove from the broiler and garnish with parsley before serving.

Nutritional Facts: Calories 263; Carbs 17.8g; Proteins 24.1g; Fat 10.6g.

41. Pork and figs mix

Prep time: 10 mins
Cooking time: 40 mins
Servings: 4
Ingredients:

- 3 Tbsp. avocado oil
- 1 and ½ lb. pork stew meat, roughly cubed
- Salt and black pepper to taste
- 1 cup red onions, chopped
- 1 cup figs, dried and chopped
- 1 Tbsp. ginger, grated
- 1 Tbsp. garlic, minced
- 1 cup canned tomatoes, crushed
- 2 Tbsp. parsley, chopped

Directions:

1. Heat up a pot with the oil over medium-high heat, add the meat and brown for 5 minutes.
2. Add the onions and sauté for 5 minutes more.
3. Add the rest of the ingredients, bring to a simmer and cook over medium heat for 30 minutes more.
4. Divide the mix between plates and serve.

Nutritional Facts: Calories 309, Fat 16g, Fiber 10.4g, Carbs 21.1g, Proteins 34.2g.

42. Steamed chicken with mushroom and ginger

Prep time: 10 mins
Cooking time: 30 mins
Servings: 4
Ingredients:

- 4 x 150g chicken breasts
- 2 tsp. extra-virgin olive oil
- 1 1/2 Tbsp. balsamic vinegar
- 8cm piece ginger, cut into matchsticks
- 1 bunch broccoli
- 1 bunch carrots, diced
- 6 small dried shiitake mushrooms, chopped
- Spring onion, sliced
- Fresh coriander leaves
- Salt and pepper

Directions:

1. In a bowl, combine the chicken with salt, vinegar, and pepper; let it marinate for at least 10 minutes.
2. Transfer the chicken to a baking dish and top with mushrooms and ginger. Cook in a preheated oven at 350 degrees for about 15 minutes.
3. Place chopped broccoli and carrots on top of the chicken and return to the oven. Cook for another 3 minutes or until chicken is tender.
4. Divide the chicken, broccoli, and carrots on serving plates and drizzle each with olive oil and top with coriander and onions. Enjoy!

Nutritional Facts: Calories 200, Fat 6.0g, Carbs 32.4g, Sugars 15.3g, Proteins 11.7g.

43. Fragrant Asian hotpot

Prep time: 10 mins
Cooking time: 20 mins
Servings: 4
Ingredients:

- 1 tsp. tomato purée
- 1 star anise, squashed (or 1/4 tsp ground anise)
- Little bunch (10g) parsley, stalks finely cleaved
- Little bunch (10g) coriander, stalks finely cleaved
- Juice of 1/2 lime
- 500ml chicken stock, new or made with 1 solid shape
- 1/2 carrot, stripped and cut into matchsticks
- 50g broccoli, cut into little florets
- 50g beansprouts
- 100 g crude tiger prawns
- 100 g firm tofu, slashed
- 50g rice noodles, cooked according to parcel directions
- 50g cooked water chestnuts, depleted
- 20g sushi ginger, slashed
- 1 Tbsp. great quality miso glue

Directions:

1. Add the tomato purée, star anise, parsley stalks, coriander stalks, lime juice and chicken stock in a pan and simmer for 10 minutes.
2. Now add the carrots, beansprouts, broccoli, prawns, tofu, noodles and water chestnuts, and cook on low heat until the prawns are cooked through.
3. Remove the pan from the stove and mix in the sushi ginger and miso glue. Serve with the parsley and coriander leaves sprinkled on top.

Nutritional Facts: Calories 434, Fat 2g, Carbs 12g, Proteins 12g, Fiber 10 g.

44. Turkey and chickpeas

Prep time: 10 mins
Cooking time: 5 hours and 10 mins
Servings: 4
Ingredients:

- 2 Tbsps. avocado oil
- 1 big turkey breast, skinless, boneless and roughly cubed
- Salt and black pepper to taste
- 1 red onion, chopped
- 15 oz. canned chickpeas, drained and rinsed
- 15 oz. canned tomatoes, chopped
- 1 cup kalamata olives, pitted and halved
- 2 Tbsp. lime juice
- 1 tsp. oregano, dried

Directions:

1. Heat the oil in a pan over medium-high heat. Add the meat and onion, and cook for 5 minutes then transfer to a slow cooker.
2. Add the rest of the ingredients, put the lid on and cook on high for 5 hours.
3. Divide between plates and serve right away!

Nutritional Facts: Calories 352, Fat 14.4g, Fiber 11.8g, Carbs 25.1g, Proteins 26.4g.

45. Beef dish

Prep time: 10 mins
Cooking time: 20 mins
Servings: 4
Ingredients:

- 1 lb. skirt steak
- 2 Tbsp. minced garlic
- 1/4 cup fresh lemon juice
- 2 Tbsp. apple cider vinegar
- 3 Tbsp. extra-virgin olive oil
- 1 tsp. salt
- 1/2 tsp. ground black pepper
- 1/4 tsp. ground cinnamon
- 1/4 tsp. ground cardamom
- 1 tsp. seven spices

Directions:

1. Using a sharp knife, cut the skirt steak into thin, 1/4-inch strips. Place the strips in a large bowl.
2. Add garlic, lemon juice, apple cider vinegar, extra-virgin olive oil, salt, black pepper, cinnamon, cardamom, and seven spices, and mix well.
3. Place the steak in the refrigerator and marinate for at least 20 minutes, and up to 24 hours.
4. Preheat a large skillet over medium heat. Add the meat and marinade, and cook for 20 minutes or until the meat is tender and the marinade has evaporated.
5. Serve warm with pita bread and tahini sauce.

Nutritional Facts: Calories 476g, Fat 40g, Fiber 9g, Carbs 33g, Proteins 6g.

46. Sesame chicken with black rice, broccoli & snap peas

Prep time: 10 mins
Cooking time: 25 mins
Servings: 4
Ingredients:

- 2/3 cup black rice
- 2 (200g each) chicken breast fillets
- 2 cups chopped broccoli
- 200g snap peas, trimmed
- 1 1/2 cups picked watercress leaves
- 1 1/2 Tbsp. salt-reduced tamari
- 1 Tbsp. sesame seeds
- 2 Tbsp. tahini
- 1/2 tsp. raw honey

Directions:

1. Boil rice in a saucepan for about 15 minutes or until al dente; then drain the excess water.
2. Coat the chicken fillets with sesame seeds and cook in hot oil in a skillet set over medium high heat for about 5 minutes per side or until cooked through.
3. Let it cool and slice.
4. In the meantime, steam the broccoli and peas until tender.
5. In a small bowl, whisk together tahini, tamari and raw honey until very smooth. Divide the cooked black rice among serving bowls and top each with broccoli, peas, chicken and watercress. Drizzle each serving with the tahini dressing. Enjoy!

Nutritional Facts: Calories: 250, Fat 15.5g, Carbs 11.5g, Sugars 3.7g, Proteins 19.2g.

47. Meatloaf

Prep time: 10 mins
Cooking time: 45 mins
Servings: 4
Ingredients:

- 2 lbs. ground beef
- 2 eggs, lightly beaten
- 1/4 tsp. dried basil
- 3 Tbsp. olive oil
- 1/2 tsp. dried sage
- 1 1/2 tsp. dried parsley
- 1 tsp. oregano
- 2 tsp. thyme
- 1 tsp. rosemary
- Salt & Pepper to taste

Directions:

1. Pour 1 1/2 cups of water into the instant pot then place the trivet in the pot.
2. Spray loaf pan with cooking spray.
3. Add all ingredients into the mixing bowl and mix until well combined.
4. Transfer meat mixture into the prepared loaf pan and place loaf pan on top of the trivet in the pot.
5. Cover the pot with the lid and cook on high for 35 minutes.
6. Once done, allow to release pressure naturally for 10 minutes and then release remaining using quick release. Remove the lid.
7. Serve and enjoy.

Nutritional Facts: Calories 365, Fat 18 g, Carbs 0.7g, Sugar 0.1g, Proteins 47.8g, Cholesterol 190mg.

CHAPTER 5:
Snacks and dessert recipes

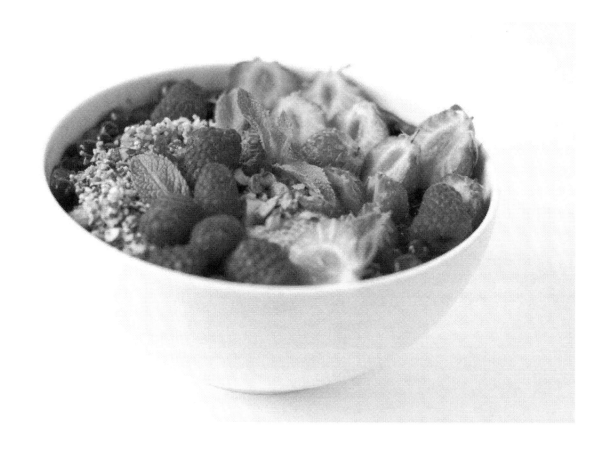

48. Minty fruit salad

Prep time: 5 mins
Cooking time: 0 mins
Servings: 4
Ingredients:

- 2 cups blueberries
- 3 Tbsp. mint, chopped
- 1 pear, cored and cubed
- 1 apple, cored, cubed
- 1 Tbsp. coconut sugar

Directions:

1. In a bowl, combine the blueberries with the mint and the other ingredients, toss, and serve cold.

Nutritional Facts: Calories 104, Proteins 1g, Carbs 26.9g, Fat 0.4g, Sodium 3mg, Potassium 175mg.

49. Dates cream

Prep time: 5 mins
Cooking time: 0 mins
Servings: 4
Ingredients:

- 1 cup almond milk
- 1 banana, peeled and sliced
- 1 tsp. vanilla extract
- ½ cup coconut cream
- 1 cup dates, chopped

Directions:

1. In a blender, combine the dates with the banana and the other ingredients, pulse well, divide into small cups and serve cold.

Nutritional Facts: Calories 119, Proteins 1.3g, Carbs 12.1g, Fat 7.9g, Sodium 40mg, Potassium 200mg.

50. Almond plum muffins

Prep time: 10 mins
Cooking time: 25 mins
Servings: 12
Ingredients:

- 3 Tbsp. coconut oil, melted
- ½ cup almond milk
- 4 eggs, whisked
- 1 tsp. vanilla extract
- 1 cup almond flour
- 2 tsp. cinnamon powder
- ½ tsp. baking powder
- 1 cup plums, pitted and chopped

Directions:

2. In a bowl, combine the coconut oil with the almond milk and the other ingredients and whisk well.
3. Divide into a muffin pan, place it in the oven at 350 degrees F and bake for 25 minutes.
4. Serve the muffins cold.

Nutritional Facts: Calories 137, Proteins 2.1g, Carbs 3.1g, Fat 12.3g, Sodium 22mg, Potassium 76mg.

51. Coconut plums bowls

Prep time: 10 mins
Cooking time: 20 mins
Servings: 4
Ingredients:

- ½ lb. plums, pitted and halved
- 2 Tbsp. coconut sugar
- 4 Tbsp. raisins
- 1 tsp. vanilla extract
- 1 cup coconut cream

Directions:

1. In a pan, combine the plums with the sugar and the other ingredients, bring to a simmer and cook over medium heat for 20 minutes.
2. Divide into bowls and serve.

Nutritional Facts: Calories 194, Proteins 1.7g, Carbs 17.6g, Fat 14.4g, Sodium 10mg, Potassium 240mg.

52. Mixed dried fruit oatmeal cookies

Prep time: 10 mins
Cooking time: 15 mins
Servings: 20
Ingredients:

- 1 1/3 cups uncooked old-fashioned oats or quick-cooking rolled oats
- 1 cup whole-wheat flour
- 1 tsp. baking powder
- 1 tsp. ground cinnamon
- ¼ tsp. ground mace
- ½ cup loosely packed brown sugar
- 1/3 cup plain low-fat yogurt
- 2 Tbsp. canola oil
- 1 egg
- 1 tsp. vanilla extract
- ½ cup mixed dried fruit
- ½ cup dark chocolate chips

Directions:

1. Preheat oven to 350°f (180°c). Line two baking sheets with baking mats or parchment paper.
2. In a medium bowl, stir together the oats, flour, baking powder, cinnamon, mace, and sugar.
3. In a large bowl, stir together yogurt, oil, egg, and vanilla. Add flour mixture to yogurt mixture. Using a spatula, mix until just combined. Stir in the dried fruit and chocolate chips.
4. Using a large spoon , drop cookie dough onto the baking sheet, about 2 inches apart.
5. Bake for 10 to 12 minutes, until lightly browned. Remove from the oven and cool on a wire rack.

Nutritional Facts: Calories 79, Fat 3g, Proteins 2g, Carbs 12g, Sodium 3mg, Potassium 91mg.

53. Walnut & spiced apple tonic

Prep time: 10 mins
Cooking time: 0 mins
Servings: 4
Ingredients:

- 6 walnuts halves
- 1 apple, cored
- 1 banana
- ½ tsp. matcha powder
- ½ tsp. cinnamon
- Pinch of ground nutmeg

Directions:

1. Place all the ingredients into a blender and add sufficient water to cover them. Blitz until smooth and creamy.

Nutritional Facts: Calories 124, Sodium 22mg, Fiber 1.4g, Fat 2.1g, Carbs 12.3g, Proteins 1.2g.

54. Raw broccoli poppers

Prep time: 10 mins
Cooking time: 10 mins
Servings: 4
Ingredients:

- 1/8 cup water
- 1/8 tsp. fine sea salt
- 4 cups broccoli florets, washed and cut into 1-inch pieces
- 1/4 tsp. turmeric powder
- 1 cup unsalted cashews, soaked overnight or at least 3-4 hours and drained
- 1/4 tsp. onion powder
- 1 red bell pepper, de-seeded and chopped
- 2 Tbsp. nutritional heaping
- 2 Tbsp. lemon juice

Directions:

2. Transfer the drained cashews to a high-speed blender and pulse for about 30 seconds. Add in the chopped pepper and pulse again for 30 seconds.
3. Add the lemon juice, water, nutritional yeast/ heaping, onion powder, sea salt, and turmeric powder. Pulse for about 45 seconds, or until smooth.
4. Take the broccoli into a bowl and add in the chopped cheesy cashew mixture. Toss well until coated.
5. Transfer the pieces of broccoli to the trays of a yeast dehydrator.
6. Follow the dehydrator's instructions and dehydrate for about 8 minutes at 125°f or until crunchy.

Nutritional Facts: Calories 408, Fat 32g, Carbs 22g, Proteins 15g.

55. Cod and cabbage

Prep time: 10 mins
Cooking time: 15 mins
Servings: 4
Ingredients:

- 3 cups green cabbage, shredded
- 1 sweet onion, sliced
- A pinch of salt and black pepper
- ½ cup feta cheese, crumbled
- 4 tsp. olive oil
- 4 cod fillets, boneless
- ¼ cup green olives, pitted and chopped

Directions:

1. Grease a roasting pan with the oil, add the fish, the cabbage and the rest of the ingredients, and cook at 450 degrees F for 15 minutes.
2. Divide the mix between plates and serve.

Nutritional Facts: Calories 270, Fat 10g, Fiber 3g, Carbs 12g, Proteins 31g.

56. Healthy carrot & shrimp

Prep time: 10 mins
Cooking time: 10 mins
Servings: 4
Ingredients:

- 1 lb. shrimp, peeled and deveined
- 1 Tbsp. chives, chopped
- 1 onion, chopped
- 1 Tbsp. olive oil
- 1 cup fish stock
- 1 cup carrots, sliced
- Pepper
- Salt

Directions:

1. Add oil into the inner pot of instant pot and set the pot on sauté mode.
2. Add onion and sauté for 2 minutes.
3. Add shrimp and stir well.
4. Add the remaining ingredients and stir well.
5. Seal the pot with lid and cook on high for 4 minutes.
6. Once done, release pressure using quick release. Remove the lid afterwards.
7. Serve and enjoy.

Nutritional Facts: Calories 197, Fat 5.9g, Carbs 7g, Sugar 2.5g, Proteins 27.7g, cholesterol 239 mg.

57. Spiced toasted almonds & seed mix

Prep time: 10 mins
Cooking time: 10 mins
Servings: 4
Ingredients:

- 2 Tbsp. olive oil
- 1/2 cup sunflower seeds
- 1/2 cup pumpkin seeds
- 1 cup almonds
- 1 Tbsp. chili paste
- 1 Tbsp. crushed fennel seeds
- 1 Tbsp. ground cumin
- ½ tsp. sea salt

Directions:

1. Heat oil in a skillet set over medium heat.
2. Stir in the chili paste and fennel seeds and then add in the other seeds and almonds.
3. Sauté for about 5 minutes and then stir in cumin and salt.
4. Remove from heat and let cool before serving.

Nutritional Facts: Calories 448, Fat 27g, Carbs 41g, Protein 15g.

58. Style nachos recipe

Prep time: 40 mins
Cooking time: 10 mins
Servings: 4
Ingredients:

- 6 pieces whole-wheat pita bread
- Cooking spray
- 1/2 tsp. ground cumin
- 1/2 tsp. ground coriander
- 1/2 tsp. paprika
- 1/2 tsp. pepper
- 1/2 tsps. salt
- 1/2 cup hot water
- 1/2 tsp. beef stock concentrate
- 1 lb. ground lamb or beef
- 2 garlic cloves, minced
- 1 tsp. cornstarch
- 2 medium cucumbers, peeled, seeded, grated
- 2 cups Greek yogurt, plain
- 2 Tbsp. lemon juice
- 1/4 tsp. grated lemon peel
- 1 tsp. salt, divided
- 1/4 tsp. pepper
- 1/2 cup pitted Greek olives, sliced
- 4 green onions, thinly sliced
- 1/2 cup crumbled feta cheese
- 2 cups torn romaine lettuce
- 2 medium tomatoes, seeded and chopped

Directions:

1. In a colander set over a bowl, toss the cucumbers with 1/2 tsp. of the salt; let stand for 30 minutes, then squeeze and pat dry. Set aside.
2. In a small-sized bowl, combine the coriander, cumin, 1/2 tsp. pepper, paprika, and 1/2 tsp. salt; set aside.
3. Cut each pita bread into 8 wedges. Arrange them in a single layer on ungreased baking sheets. Spritz both sides of the wedges with cooking spray. Sprinkle with 3/4 tsp. of the seasoning mix. Broil 3-4 inches from the heat source for about 3-4 minutes per side, or until golden brown. Transfer to wire racks, let cool.

4. Whisk hot water and beef stock cube in a liquid measuring cup until blended. In a large-sized skillet, cook the lamb, seasoned with the remaining seasoning mix, over medium heat until the meat is no longer pink. Add the garlic; cook for 1 minute. Drain.
5. Stir in the cornstarch into the broth; mix until smooth. Gradually stir into the skillet; bring to a boil and cook, stirring, for 2 minutes or until thick.
6. In a small-sized bowl, combine the cucumbers, yogurt, lemon peel, lemon juice, and the remaining salt and pepper.
7. Arrange the pita wedges on a serving platter. Layer with the lettuce, lamb mixture, tomatoes, onions, olives, and cheese; serve immediately with the cucumber sauce.

Nutritional Facts: Calories 232, Fat 6.7g, Cholesterol 42mg, Sodium 630mg, Carbs 24, Fiber 3.3g, Sugar 4.1g, Proteins 20.2g.

59. Basil tilapia

Prep time: 10 mins
Cooking time: 20 mins
Servings: 4
Ingredients:

- 12 oz. tilapia fillet
- 2 oz. parmesan, grated
- 1 Tbsp. olive oil
- ½ tsp. ground black pepper
- 1 cup fresh basil
- 3 Tbsp. avocado oil
- 1 Tbsp. pine nuts
- 1 garlic clove, peeled
- ¾ tsp. white pepper

Directions:

1. Make pesto sauce: blend the avocado oil, fresh basil, pine nuts, garlic cloves, and white pepper until smooth.
2. After this, cut the tilapia fillet into 3 servings.
3. Sprinkle every fish serving with olive oil and ground black pepper.
4. Roast the fillets over medium heat for 2 minutes on each side.
5. Meanwhile, line the baking tray with baking paper.
6. Arrange the roasted tilapia fillets in the tray.
7. Then top them with pesto and parmesan.
8. Bake the fish for 15 minutes at 365f.
9. Drizzle the sauce on top and serve.

Nutritional Facts: Calories 321, Fat 17g, Fiber 1.2g, Carbs 4.4g, Proteins 37.4g.

60. Marinated cheese

Prep time: 10 mins
Cooking time: 10 mins
Servings: 4
Ingredients:

- 8 oz. cream cheese
- 6 sprigs fresh thyme
- 3 sprigs fresh rosemary
- 2 garlic cloves, sliced
- 1/2 cup sun-dried tomato vinaigrette dressing
- 1 tsp. black pepper
- 1 lemon peel, cut into thin strips

Directions:

1. Cut the cream cheese into 36 cubes. Place on a serving tray.
2. Combine the remaining ingredients together.
3. Pour the dressing over the cheese; toss lightly.
4. Refrigerate for at least 1 hour before serving.

Nutritional Facts: Calories 44, Fat 4.3g, Cholesterol 13.9mg, Sodium 40.6mg, Carbs 0.7g , Proteins 0.8g.

61. Savory pita chips

Prep time: 10 mins
Cooking time: 10 mins
Servings: 4
Ingredients:

- 3 pitas
- 1/4 cup extra-virgin olive oil
- 1/4 cup zaatar

Directions:

1. Preheat the oven to 450ºF.
2. Cut pitas into 2-inch pieces, and place in a large bowl.
3. Drizzle pitas with extra-virgin olive oil, sprinkle with zaatar, and toss to coat.
4. Spread out pitas on a baking sheet, and bake for 8 to 10 minutes or until lightly browned and crunchy.
5. Let pita chips cool before removing from the baking sheet. Store in an airtight container for up to 1 month.

Nutritional Facts: Calories 242, Carbs 25g, Fat 12g, Proteins 13g.

62. Carrot chips

Prep time: 10 mins
Cooking time: 20 mins
Servings: 4
Ingredients:

- 6 large carrots
- 2 Tbsp. extra virgin olive oil
- ½ tsp. black pepper

Directions:

1. Chop the carrots into 2-inch sections and then cut each section into thin sticks.
2. Toss together the carrots sticks with extra virgin olive oil and pepper in a bowl and spread onto a baking sheet lined with parchment paper.
3. Bake the carrot sticks at 425° for about 20 minutes or until browned.

Nutrition: Calories 448, Fat 27g, Carbs 41g, Proteins 15g.

63. Roasted radishes

Prep time: 10 mins
Cooking time: 35 mins
Servings: 4
Ingredients:

- 2 cups radishes cut in quarters
- Salt and ground black pepper to taste
- 2 Tbsp. butter, melted
- 1 Tbsp. fresh chives, chopped
- 1 Tbsp. lemon zest

Directions:

1. Spread the radishes on a lined baking sheet. Add the salt, pepper, chives, lemon zest, and butter, toss to coat, and bake in the oven at 375°F for 35 minutes.
2. Divide onto plates and serve.

Nutrition: Calories 122, Fat 12 g, Carbs 3 g, Proteins 14 g.

64. Superfood raw bars

Prep time: 10 mins
Cooking time: 5 mins
Servings: 4
Ingredients:

- 1 /2 cup toasted pistachios
- 1/4 cup goji berries + 2 Tbsp. more
- 1 /2 cup roasted almonds
- 1/4 cup chia seeds
- 3 /4 cup blackcurrants
- 3 /4 cup coconut flakes, toasted
- 1 /3 cup ginger
- 1 Tbsp. raw cacao nibs
- 1 Tbsp. coconut oil
- 500g chopped dark chocolate
- Pinch of sea salt

Directions:

1. Prepare a baking pan by greasing and lining with baking paper.
2. In a large bowl, combine 1/3 cup of pistachios, blackcurrants, ½ cup of coconut flakes, goji berries, almond, chia pieces, and ginger until well mixed.
3. In another bowl, stir together cacao nibs, the remaining pistachios and coconut flakes, and more goji berries.
4. In a saucepan, stir together oil, chocolate and salt until the chocolate is melted. Pour the chocolate mixture into the pistachio mixture and stir until well coated; transfer to the pan and sprinkle with the cacao mixture.
5. Refrigerate for at least 4 hours or until firm. Cut into 24 squares and serve, storing the rest in the refrigerator for up two weeks.

Nutritional Facts: Calories 448, Fat 27g, Carbs 41g, Proteins 15g.

65. Cheese rolls

Prep time: 10 mins
Cooking time: 10 mins
Servings: 4
Ingredients:

- 1 cup ackawi cheese
- 1 cup shredded mozzarella cheese
- 2 Tbsp. fresh parsley, finely chopped
- 1 large egg
- 1/2 tsp. ground black pepper
- 1 large egg yolk, beaten
- 2 Tbsp. Water
- 1 pkg. egg roll dough (20 count)
- 4 Tbsp. extra-virgin olive oil

Directions:

1. In a large bowl, combine ackawi cheese, mozzarella cheese, parsley, egg, and black pepper.
2. In a separate bowl, whisk together egg yolk and water.
3. Lay out 1 egg roll, place 2 Tbsp. cheese mixture at one corner of the roll, and brush the opposite corner with the egg yolk mixture.
4. Fold over the side of the egg roll with cheese to the middle. Fold in the left and right sides, and complete rolling the egg roll using the egg-brushed side to seal. Set aside, seal side down, and repeat with the remaining egg rolls and cheese mixture.
5. In a skillet over low heat, heat 2 Tbsp. extra-virgin olive oil. Add up to 4 cheese rolls, seal side down, and cook for 1 or 2 minutes per side or until browned. Repeat with remaining 2 Tbsps. extra-virgin olive oil and egg rolls.
6. Serve warm.

Nutritional Facts: Calories 242, Carbs 25g, Fat 12g, Proteins 13g.

66. Chia crackers

Prep time: 10 mins
Cooking time: 30 mins
Servings: 4
Ingredients:

- 1/2 cup pecans, chopped
- 1/2 cup chia seeds
- 1/2 tsp. cayenne pepper
- 1 cup water
- 1/4 cup nutritional yeast
- 1/2 cup pumpkin seeds
- 1/4 cup ground flax
- Salt and pepper, to taste

Directions:

1. Mix around 1/2 cup of chia seeds and 1 cup of water. Keep it aside.
2. Take another bowl and combine all the remaining ingredients. Combine well and stir in the chia water mixture until you obtain a dough.
3. Transfer the dough onto a baking sheet and roll it out into a ¼"-thick dough.
4. Transfer into a preheated oven at 325ºf and bake for about ½ hour.
5. Take out from the oven, flip over the dough, and cut it into desired cracker shaped-squares.
6. Spread and back again for a further half an hour, or until crispy and browned.
7. Once done, take them out from the oven and let them cool at room temperature. Enjoy!

Nutritional Facts: Calories 41, Fats 3.1g, Carbs 2g, Proteins 2g.

67. Chili mango and watermelon salsa

Prep time: 10 mins
Cooking time: 0 mins
Servings: 4
Ingredients:

- 1 red tomato, chopped
- Salt and black pepper to taste
- 1 cup watermelon, seedless, peeled and cubed
- 1 red onion, chopped
- 2 mangos, peeled and chopped
- 2 chili peppers, chopped
- ¼ cup cilantro, chopped
- 3 Tbsp. lime juice
- Pita chips for serving

Directions:

1. In a bowl, mix the tomato with the watermelon, onion and the rest of the ingredients except the pita chips, and toss well.
2. Divide the mix into small cups and serve with pita chips on the side.

Nutritional Facts: Calories 62, Fat 4.7g, Fiber 1.3g, Carbs 3.9g, Proteins 2.3g.

68. Healthy guacamole

Prep time: 10 mins
Cooking time: 0 mins
Servings: 4
Ingredients:

- 2 medium ripe avocados, peeled, pitted and chopped
- 1 small red onion, chopped
- 1 garlic clove, minced
- 1 serrano pepper, seeded and chopped
- 1 tomato, seeded and chopped
- 2 Tbsp. fresh cilantro leaves, chopped
- 1 Tbsp. fresh lime juice
- Salt, to taste

Directions:

1. In a large bowl, add avocado and, with a fork, mash it completely.
2. Add all the remaining ingredients and gently stir to combine.
3. Serve immediately.

Nutritional Facts: Calories 448, Fat 27g, Carbs 41g, Proteins 15g.

69. Healthy spinach dip

Prep time: 10 mins
Cooking time: 15 mins
Servings: 4
Ingredients:

- 14 oz. spinach
- 2 Tbsp. fresh lime juice
- 1 Tbsp. garlic, minced
- 2 Tbsp. olive oil
- 2 Tbsp. coconut cream
- Pepper
- Salt

Directions:

1. Add all ingredients except coconut cream into the instant pot and stir well.
2. Seal the pot with lid and cook on low pressure for 8 minutes.
3. Once done, allow to release pressure naturally for 5 minutes then release remaining using quick release. Remove lid.
4. Add coconut cream and stir well and blend spinach mixture using a blender until smooth.
5. Serve and enjoy.

Nutritional Facts: Calories 109, Fat 9.2g, Carbs 6.6g, Sugar 1.1g, Proteins 3.2g, Cholesterol 0 mg.

70. Lavash roll ups

Prep time: 10 mins
Cooking time: 0 mins
Servings: 4
Ingredients:

- 2 lavash wraps (whole-wheat)
- 1/4 cup roasted red peppers, sliced
- 1/4 cup black olives, sliced
- 1/2 cup hummus of choice
- 1/2 cup grape tomatoes, halved
- 1 medium cucumber, sliced
- Fresh dill, for garnish

Directions:

1. Lay out the lavash wraps on a clean surface. Evenly spread hummus over each piece.
2. Layer the cucumbers across the wraps, about 1/2-inch from each other, leaving about 2-icnh empty space at the bottom of the wrap for rolling purposes.
3. Place the roasted pepper slices around the cucumbers. Sprinkle with black olives and the tomatoes. Garnish with freshly chopped dill.
4. Tightly roll each wrap, using the hummus at the end to almost glue the wrap into a roll.
5. Slice each roll into 4 equal pieces. Secure each piece by sticking a toothpick through the center of each roll slice.
6. Lay each on a serving bowl or tray; garnish with fresh dill.

Nutritional Facts: Calories 250, Total Fat 8g, Saturated Fat 0.5g, Cholesterol 0mg, Sodium 440mg, Potassium 340mg, Carbs 43g, Fiber 40g, Sugar 3g, Proteins 10g.

71. Rosemary & garlic kale chips

Prep time: 10 mins
Cooking time: 30 mins
Servings: 4
Ingredients:

- 9oz kale chips, chopped into 2-inch pieces
- 2 sprigs of rosemary
- 2 cloves of garlic
- 2 Tbsp. olive oil
- Sea salt
- Freshly ground black pepper

Directions:

1. Gently warm the olive oil, rosemary and garlic over a low heat for 10 minutes. Remove it from the heat and set aside to cool.
2. Take the rosemary and garlic out of the oil and discard them.
3. Toss the kale leaves in the oil, making sure they are well coated.
4. Season with salt and pepper.
5. Spread the kale leaves onto 2 baking sheets and bake them in the oven at 170 C/325 For 15 minutes, until crispy.

Nutritional Facts: Calories 249, Sodium 36mg, Fiber 1.7g, Fat 4.3g, Carbs 15.3g, Proteins 1.4g.

72. Pepper salmon skewers

Prep time: 30 mins
Cooking time: 20 mins
Servings: 4
Ingredients:

- 1.5-lb. salmon fillet
- ½ cup plain yogurt
- 1 tsp. paprika
- 1 tsp. turmeric
- 1 tsp. red pepper
- 1 tsp. salt
- 1 tsp. dried cilantro
- 1 tsp. sunflower oil
- ½ tsp. ground nutmeg

Directions:

1. For the marinade: mix together the plain yogurt, paprika, turmeric, red pepper, salt, and ground nutmeg.
2. Chop the salmon fillet roughly and put it in the yogurt mixture.
3. Mix up well and marinate for 25 minutes.
4. Then skew the fish on the skewers.
5. Sprinkle the skewers with sunflower oil and place in the tray.
6. Bake the salmon skewers for 15 minutes at 375F.
7. Season with the cilantro and serve hot.

Nutritional Facts: Calories 217, Fat 9.9g, Fiber 0.6g, Carbs 4.2g, Proteins 28.1g.

73. Garlic mussels

Prep time: 10 mins
Cooking time: 10 mins
Servings: 4
Ingredients:

- 1-lb. mussels
- 1 chili pepper, chopped
- 1 cup chicken stock
- ½ cup milk
- 1 tsp. olive oil
- 1 tsp. minced garlic
- 1 tsp. ground coriander
- ½ tsp. salt
- 1 cup fresh parsley, chopped
- 4 Tbsp. lemon juice

Directions:

1. Pour milk in the saucepan.
2. Add chili pepper, chicken stock, olive oil, minced garlic, ground coriander, salt, and lemon juice.
3. Bring the liquid to boil and add mussels.
4. Boil the mussel for 4 minutes or until they will open shells.
5. Then add chopped parsley and mix up the meal well.
6. Remove it from the heat.

Nutritional Facts: Calories 136, Fat 4.7g, Fiber 0.6g, Carbs 7.5g, Proteins 15.3g.

74. Superfood spiced apricot-sesame bliss balls

Prep time: 10 mins
Cooking time: 0 mins
Servings: 4
Ingredients:

- 2 Tbsps. sesame seeds
- 1 cup apricots
- 1 cup natural gluten-free muesli
- 1 cup almonds
- 2 Tbsp. raw honey
- 1 tsp. ground cinnamon

Directions:

1. In a food processor, process almonds until finely chopped; add in raw honey, muesli, apricots, and cinnamon and process until very smooth.
2. Add sesame seeds in a shallow dish. Roll two Tbsp. of the almond mixture into bite-sized balls and then roll them into the sesame seeds until well coated.
3. Arrange them on a tray and refrigerate until set. Serve and store the rest in an airtight container.

Nutritional Facts: Calories 448, Fat 27g, Carbs 41g, Proteins 15g.

75. Halibut and quinoa mix

Prep time: 10 mins
Cooking time: 10 mins
Servings: 4
Ingredients:

- 4 halibut fillets, boneless
- 2 Tbsp. olive oil
- 1 tsp. rosemary, dried
- 2 tsp. cumin, ground
- 1 Tbsp. coriander, ground
- 2 tsp. cinnamon powder
- 2 tsp. oregano, dried
- A pinch of salt and black pepper
- 2 cups quinoa, cooked
- 1 cup cherry tomatoes, halved
- 1 avocado, peeled, pitted and sliced
- 1 cucumber, cubed
- ½ cup black olives, pitted and sliced
- Juice of 1 lemon

Directions:

1. In a bowl, combine the fish with the rosemary, cumin, coriander, cinnamon, oregano, salt and pepper and toss.
2. Heat up a pan with the oil over medium heat, add the fish, and sear for 2 minutes on each side.
3. Introduce the pan in the oven and bake the fish at 425 degrees f for 7 minutes.
4. Meanwhile, in a bowl, mix the quinoa with the remaining ingredients, toss and divide between plates.
5. Add the fish next to the quinoa mix and serve right away.

Nutritional Facts: Calories 364, Fat 15.4g, Fiber 11.2g, Carbs 56.4g, Proteins 24.5g.

76. Orange-spiced pumpkin hummus

Prep time: 10 mins
Cooking time: 0 mins
Servings: 4
Ingredients:

- 1 Tbsp. maple syrup
- 1/2 tsp. salt
- 1 can (16 oz.) Garbanzo beans
- 1/8 tsp. ginger or nutmeg
- 1 cup canned pumpkin blend
- 1/8 tsp. cinnamon
- 1/4 cup tahini
- 1 Tbsp. fresh orange juice
- Pinch of orange zest, for garnish
- 1 Tbsp. apple cider vinegar

Directions:

1. Mix all the ingredients in a food processor or blender until slightly chunky.
2. Serve right away, and enjoy!

Nutritional Facts: Calories 291, Fats 22.9g, Carbs 15g, Proteins 12g.

77. Artichoke skewers

Prep time: 10 mins
Cooking time: 10 mins
Servings: 4
Ingredients:

- 4 prosciutto slices
- 4 artichoke hearts, canned
- 4 kalamata olives
- 4 cherry tomatoes
- ¼ tsp. cayenne pepper
- ¼ tsp. sunflower oil

Directions:

1. Skewer prosciutto slices, artichoke hearts, kalamata olives, and cherry tomatoes on the wooden skewers.
2. Sprinkle antipasti skewers with sunflower oil and cayenne pepper.

Nutritional Facts: Calories 152, Fat 3.7g, Fiber 10.8g, Carbs 23.2g, Proteins 11.1g.

CHAPTER 6:
Dinner recipes

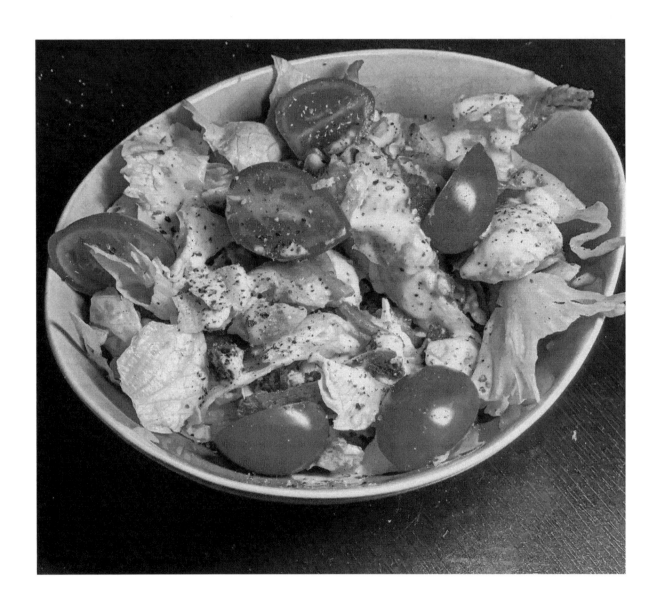

78. Delicious lemon chicken salad

Prep time: 15 mins
Cooking time: 5 mins
Servings: 4
Ingredients:

- 1 lb. Chicken breast, cooked and diced
- 1 Tbsp. fresh dill, chopped
- 2 tsp. olive oil
- 1/4 cup low-fat yogurt
- 1 tsp. lemon zest, grated
- 2 Tbsp. onion, minced
- ¼ tsp. pepper
- ¼ tsp. salt

Directions:

1. Put all your ingredients into a large mixing bowl and toss well. Season with pepper and salt. Cover and place in the refrigerator. Serve chilled and enjoy.

Nutritional Facts: Calories 165, Fat 5.4g, Proteins 25.2g, Carbs 2.2g, Sodium 153mg.

79. Healthy chicken orzo

Prep time: 15 mins
Cooking time: 15 mins
Servings: 4
Ingredients:

- 1 cup whole wheat orzo
- 1 lb. chicken breasts, sliced
- ½ tsp. red pepper flakes
- ½ cup feta cheese, crumbled
- ½ tsp. oregano
- 1 Tbsp. fresh parsley, chopped
- 1 Tbsp. fresh basil, chopped
- ¼ cup pine nuts
- 1 cup spinach, chopped
- ¼ cup white wine
- ½ cup olives, sliced
- 1 cup grape tomatoes, cut in half
- ½ Tbsp. garlic, minced
- 2 Tbsp. olive oil
- ½ tsp. pepper
- ½ tsp. salt

Directions:

2. Heat 1 Tbsp. of olive oil in a pan over medium heat. Season chicken with pepper and salt and cook in the pan for 5-7 minutes on each side. Remove from the pan and set aside.
3. Add water in a small saucepan and bring to boil. Add orzo in the boiling water and cook according to the packet directions. Heat the remaining olive oil in a pan on medium heat, then put garlic in the pan and sauté for a minute. Stir in white wine and cherry tomatoes and cook on high for 3 minutes.
4. Add cooked orzo, spices, spinach, pine nuts, and olives and stir until well combined. Add chicken on top of orzo and sprinkle with feta cheese. Serve and enjoy.

Nutritional Facts: Calories 518, Fat 27.7g, Proteins 40.6g, Carbs 26.2g, Sodium 121mg.

80. Lemon garlic chicken

Prep time: 15 mins
Cooking time: 12 mins
Servings: 3
Ingredients:

- 3 chicken breasts, cut into thin slices
- 2 lemon zest, grated
- ¼ cup olive oil
- 4 garlic cloves, minced
- Pepper
- Salt

Directions:

1. Warm-up olive oil in a pan over medium heat. Add garlic to the pan and sauté for 30 seconds.
2. Put the chicken in the pan and sauté within 10 minutes.
3. Add lemon zest and lemon juice and bring to boil.
4. Remove from heat and season with pepper and salt. Serve and enjoy.

Nutritional Facts: Calories 439, Fat 27.8g, Proteins 42.9g, Carbs 4.9g, Sodium 306mg.

81. Chicken cacciatore

Prep time: 5 mins
Cooking time: 45 mins
Servings: 6
Ingredients:

- 2 Tbsp. extra virgin olive oil
- 6 chicken thighs
- 1 sweet onion, chopped
- 2 garlic cloves, minced
- 2 red bell peppers, cored and diced
- 2 carrots, diced
- 1 rosemary sprig
- 1 thyme sprig
- 4 tomatoes, peeled and diced
- ½ cup tomato juice
- ¼ cup dry white wine
- 1 cup chicken stock
- 1 bay leaf
- Salt and pepper to taste

Directions:

1. Heat the oil in a heavy saucepan.
2. Cook chicken on all sides until golden.
3. Stir in the onion and garlic and cook for 2 minutes.
4. Stir in the rest of the ingredients and season with salt and pepper.
5. Cook on low heat for 30 minutes.
6. Serve the chicken cacciatore warm and fresh.

Nutritional Facts: Calories 363, Fat 14g, Proteins 42g, Carbs 9g.

82. Fennel wild rice risotto

Prep time: 5 mins
Cooking time: 35 mins
Servings: 6
Ingredients:

- 2 Tbsp. extra virgin olive oil
- 1 shallot, chopped
- 2 garlic cloves, minced
- 1 fennel bulb, chopped
- 1 cup wild rice
- ¼ cup dry white wine
- 2 cups chicken stock
- 1 tsp. grated orange zest
- Salt and pepper to taste

Directions:

1. Heat the oil in a heavy saucepan.
2. Add the garlic, shallot and fennel and cook for a few minutes until softened.
3. Stir in the rice and cook for 2 additional minutes then add the wine, stock and orange zest, with salt and pepper to taste.
4. Cook on low heat for 20 minutes.
5. Serve the risotto warm and fresh.

Nutritional Facts: Calories 162, Fat 2g, Proteins 8g, Carbs 20g.

83. Brazilian-inspired shrimp stew

Prep time: 10 mins
Cooking time: 20 mins
Servings: 4
Ingredients:

- 1 ½ lb. jumbo shrimp, peeled and deveined
- 2 cloves garlic, minced
- ¼ cup olive oil
- 1 small yellow onion, diced
- ¼ cup fresh cilantro, chopped
- ¼ cup roasted red peppers, diced
- 1 (14 oz.) can chopped tomatoes with chilies
- 2 Tbsp. sambal oelek – check in the Asian food section in the supermarket or food store
- 1 cup full-fat coconut milk
- Juice of 1 lime
- Freshly ground pepper and sea salt to taste

Directions:

1. Pour the olive oil in a saucepan over medium to high heat and sauté the onions until tender.
2. Stir in the roasted peppers and garlic and cook until fragrant, careful not to burn the garlic.
3. Stir in the shrimp, tomatoes and three quarter of the cilantro. Cook until the shrimp turns opaque for 5-8 minutes.
4. Stir in the sambal oelek and pour in the coconut milk. Reduce heat to low and cook for 5 minutes then add the lime juice and season well with pepper and salt.
5. Turn of the heat and garnish with the extra cilantro and serve hot.

Nutritional Facts: Calories 390, Fat 9g, Carbs 23g, Proteins 7g.

84. Cardamom chicken and apricot sauce

Prep time: 10 mins
Cooking time: 7 hours
Servings: 4
Ingredients:

- Juice of ½ lemon
- Zest of ½ lemon, grated
- 2 tsp. cardamom, ground
- Salt and black pepper to the taste
- 2 chicken breasts, skinless, boneless and halved
- 2 Tbsp. olive oil
- 2 spring onions, chopped
- 2 Tbsp. tomato paste
- 2 garlic cloves, minced
- 1 cup apricot juice
- ½ cup chicken stock
- ¼ cup cilantro, chopped

Directions:

1. In your slow cooker, combine the chicken with the lemon juice, lemon zest and the other ingredients except the cilantro, toss, put the lid on and cook on low for 7 hours.
2. Divide the mix between plates, sprinkle the cilantro on top and serve.

Nutritional Facts: Calories 323, Fat 12g, Fiber 11g, Carbs 23.8g, Proteins 16.4g.

85. Chicken and spinach cakes

Prep time: 10 mins
Cooking time: 15 mins
Servings: 4
Ingredients:

- 8 oz. ground chicken
- 1 cup fresh spinach, blended
- 1 tsp. minced garlic
- ½ tsp. salt
- 1 red bell pepper, grinded
- 1 egg, beaten
- 1 tsp. ground black pepper
- 4 Tbsp. panko breadcrumbs

Directions:

1. In a mixing bowl, mix together the ground chicken, blended spinach, minced garlic, salt, grinded bell pepper, egg, and ground black pepper.
2. When the chicken mixture is smooth, make 4 burgers from it and coat them in panko breadcrumbs.
3. Place the burgers in a non-sticky baking dish or line the baking tray with baking paper.
4. Bake the burgers for 15 minutes at 365F.
5. Flip the chicken burgers after 7 minutes of cooking.

Nutritional Facts: Calories 171g, Fat 5.7g, Fiber 1.7g, Carbs 10.5g, Proteins 19.4g.

86. Fragrant Asian hotpot

Prep time: 10 mins
Cooking time: 20 mins
Servings: 2
Ingredients:

- 1 tsp. tomato purée
- 1 star anise, squashed (or 1/4 tsp ground anise)
- Little bunch (10g) parsley, stalks finely cleaved
- Little bunch (10g) coriander, stalks finely cleaved
- Juice of 1/2 lime
- 500ml chicken stock, new or made with 1 solid shape
- 1/2 carrot, stripped and cut into matchsticks
- 50g broccoli, cut into little florets
- 50g beansprouts
- 100g crude tiger prawns
- 100g firm tofu, slashed
- 50g rice noodles, cooked according to parcel directions
- 50g cooked water chestnuts, depleted
- 20g sushi ginger, slashed
- 1 Tbsp. great quality miso glue

Directions:

1. Add the tomato purée, star anise, parsley stalks, coriander stalks, lime juice and chicken stock in a pan and stew for 10 minutes.
2. Now add the carrot, broccoli, beansprouts, prawns, tofu, noodles and water chestnuts, and stew tenderly until the prawns are cooked through.
3. Turn off the flame and mix in the sushi ginger and miso glue. Serve sprinkled with the parsley and coriander leaves.

Nutritional Facts: Calories 434, Fat 2g, Carbs 12g, Proteins 12g, Fiber 6g.

87. Lemon chicken mix

Prep time: 10 mins
Cooking time: 10 mins
Servings: 4
Ingredients:

- 8 oz. chicken breast, skinless, boneless
- 1 tsp. Cajun seasoning
- 1 tsp. balsamic vinegar
- 1 tsp. olive oil
- 1 tsp. lemon juice

Directions:

1. Cut the chicken breast into halves and sprinkle with Cajun seasoning, olive oil, balsamic vinegar and lemon juice.
2. Preheat the grill to 385 degrees F.
3. Grill the chicken breast halves for 5 minutes from each side.
4. Slice the Cajun chicken and place in the serving plate.

Nutritional Facts: Calories 150, Fat 5.2g, Fiber 8g, Carbs 0.1g, Proteins 24.1g.

88. Mustard chops with apricot-basil relish

Prep time: 10 mins
Cooking time: 15 mins
Servings: 4
Ingredients:

- ¼ cup basil, finely shredded
- ¼ cup olive oil
- ½ cup mustard
- ¾ lb. fresh apricots, stone removed, and fruit diced
- 1 shallot, diced small
- 1 tsp. ground cardamom
- 3 Tbsp. raspberry vinegar
- 4 pork chops
- Pepper and salt to taste

Directions:

1. Make sure that pork chops are defrosted well. Season with pepper and salt. Slather both sides of each pork chop with mustard. Preheat grill to medium-high fire.
2. In a medium bowl, mix cardamom, olive oil, vinegar, basil, shallots, and apricots. Toss to combine and season with pepper and salt, mixing once again.
3. Grill chops for 5 to 6 minutes per side. As you flip, baste with mustard.
4. Serve the pork chops with the apricot-basil relish and enjoy.

Nutritional Facts: Calories 486.5; Carbs 7.3g; Proteins 42.1g; Fat 32.1g.

89. Pepper chicken and lettuce wraps

Prep time: 10 mins
Cooking time: 10 mins
Servings: 4
Ingredients:

- 450g lean diced chicken
- 1 Tbsp. extra-virgin olive oil
- 1 tsp. black pepper
- 1 tsp. white pepper
- 1 tsp. salt
- 1 cup bean sprouts, trimmed
- 16 baby cos lettuce leaves
- 1 large red onion, diced
- 12 fresh lemon wedges
- 16 large fresh mint leaves

Directions:

1. Preheat your pan over medium high heat. In a bowl, mix together oil, white pepper, salt and black pepper until well combined; add in chicken and toss to coat well. Grill for about 5 minutes per side or until cooked through. Let rest for at least 5 minutes.
2. Arrange lettuce leaves on serving plates and top each with mint, onions and bean sprouts. Serve topped with the chicken and garnished with lemon wedges.

Nutritional Facts: Calories 381, Fat 28.5g, Carbs 30.8g, proteins 6.4g.

90. Saffron beef

Prep time: 10 mins
Cooking time: 15 mins
Servings: 4
Ingredients:

- ¾ tsp. saffron
- ¾ tsp. dried thyme
- ¾ tsp. ground coriander
- ¼ tsp. ground cinnamon
- 1 Tbsp. butter
- 1/3 tsp. salt
- 9 oz. beef sirloin

Directions:

1. Rub the beef sirloin with dried thyme, ground coriander, saffron, ground cinnamon, and salt.
2. Leave the meat for at least 10 minutes to soak all the spices.
3. Then preheat the grill to 395 degrees F.
4. Place the beef sirloin in the grill and cook it for 5 minutes.
5. Then spread the meat with butter carefully and cook for 10 minutes more. Flip it from time to time.

Nutritional Facts: Calories 291, Fat 13.8g, Fiber 0.3g, Carbs 0.6g, Proteins 38.8g.

91. Stewed chicken Greek style

Prep time: 10 mins
Cooking time: 60 mins
Servings: 4
Ingredients:

- ½ cup red wine
- 1 ½ cups chicken stock or more if needed
- 1 cup olive oil
- 1 cup tomato sauce
- 1 pc or 4lbs whole chicken cut into pieces
- 1 pinch dried oregano or to taste
- 10 small shallots, peeled
- 2 bay leaves
- 2 cloves garlic, finely chopped
- 2 Tbsp. chopped fresh parsley
- 2 tsp. butter
- Salt and ground black pepper to taste

Directions:

1. Bring to a boil a large pot of lightly salted water. Mix in the shallots and let boil uncovered until tender for around three minutes. Then drain the shallots and dip in cold water until they are no longer warm.
2. In another large pot over medium fire, heat butter and olive oil until bubbling and melted. Then sauté in the chicken and shallots for 15 minutes or until the chicken is cooked and shallots are soft and translucent. Then add the chopped garlic and cook for three mins more.
3. Then add bay leaves, oregano, salt and pepper, parsley, tomato sauce and the red wine and let simmer for a minute before adding the chicken stock. Stir before covering and let cook for 50 minutes on medium-low fire. Add the chicken and serve hot.

Nutritional Facts: Calories 644.8; Carbs 8.2g; Proteins 62.1g; Fat 40.4g.

92. Vegetable lover's chicken soup

Prep time: 10 mins
Cooking time: 20 mins
Servings: 4
Ingredients:

- 1 ½ cups baby spinach
- 2 Tbsp. orzo (tiny pasta)
- ¼ cup dry white wine
- 1 14oz. low-sodium chicken broth
- 2 plum tomatoes, chopped
- 1/8 tsp. salt
- ½ tsp. Italian seasoning
- 1 large shallot, chopped
- 1 small zucchini, diced
- 8-oz. chicken tenders
- 1 Tbsp. extra virgin olive oil

Directions:

1. In a large saucepan, heat oil over medium heat and add the chicken. Stir occasionally for 8 minutes or until browned. Transfer in a plate. Set aside.
2. In the same saucepan, add the zucchini, Italian seasoning, shallot and salt, and stir often until the vegetables are softened, around 4 minutes.
3. Add the tomatoes, wine, broth and orzo and increase the heat to high to bring the mixture to boil. Reduce the heat and simmer.
4. Add the cooked chicken and stir in the spinach last.
5. Serve hot.

Nutritional Facts: Calories 207; Carbs 14.8g; Proteins 12.2g; Fat 11.4g.

93. Wild rice prawn salad

Prep time: 5 mins
Cooking time: 35 mins
Servings: 6
Ingredients:

- ¾ cup wild rice
- 1¾ cups chicken stock
- 1 lb. prawns
- Salt and pepper to taste
- 2 Tbsp. lemon juice
- 2 Tbsp. extra virgin olive oil
- 2 cups arugula

Directions:

1. Combine the rice and chicken stock in a saucepan and cook until the liquid has been absorbed entirely.
2. Transfer the rice in a salad bowl.
3. Season the prawns with salt and pepper and drizzle them with lemon juice and oil.
4. Heat a grill pan over medium flame.
5. Place the prawns on the hot pan and cook on each side for 2-3 minutes.
6. For the salad, combine the rice with arugula and prawns and mix well.
7. Serve the salad fresh.

Nutritional Facts: Calories 207, Fat 4g, Proteins 20.6g, Carbs 17g.

94. Tasty lamb ribs

Prep time: 10 mins
Cooking time: 2 hours
Servings: 4
Ingredients:

- 2 garlic cloves, minced
- ¼ cup shallot, chopped
- 2 Tbsp. fish sauce
- ½ cup veggie stock
- 2 Tbsp. olive oil
- 1 and ½ Tbsp. lemon juice
- 1 Tbsp. coriander seeds, ground
- 1 Tbsp. ginger, grated
- Salt and black pepper to the taste
- 2 lb. lamb ribs

Directions:

1. In a roasting pan, combine the lamb with all the other ingredients. Toss them together until combined well.
2. Place it in the oven at 300 degrees F and cook for 2 hours.
3. Divide the lamb between plates and serve with a side salad.

Nutritional Facts: Calories 293, Fat 9.1g, Fiber 9.6g, Carbs 16.7g, Proteins 24.2g.

95. Simple sautéed spinach

Prep time: 10 mins
Cooking time: 6 mins
Servings: 4
Ingredients:

- 1/4 tsp. crushed red pepper
- 4 cloves garlic, thinly sliced
- 2 Tbsps. extra-virgin olive oil
- 20 oz. fresh spinach
- 1/4 tsp. low sodium salt
- 1 Tbsp. lemon juice

Directions:

1. Heat oil on medium heat in a Dutch oven.
2. Add in the garlic and cook until lightly brown (about 1 minute).
3. Stir in the spinach. Cover and cook until the spinach wilts (about 5 minutes).
4. Remove from the heat and add in salt, crushed red pepper and lemon juice.
5. Toss and serve immediately.

Nutritional Facts: Calories 118, Fat 4g, Fiber 12g, Carbs 12.7g, Proteins 19.2g.

96. Lamb chops

Prep time: 30 mins
Cooking time: 10 mins
Servings: 4
Ingredients:

- 6 (3/4-in.-thick) lamb chops
- 2 Tbsp. fresh rosemary, finely chopped
- 3 Tbsp. minced garlic
- 1 tsp. salt
- 1 tsp. ground black pepper
- 3 Tbsp. extra-virgin olive oil

Directions:

1. In a large bowl, combine the lamb chops, rosemary, garlic, salt, black pepper, and extra-virgin olive oil until the chops are evenly coated. Let them marinate at room temperature for at least 25 minutes.
2. Preheat a grill to medium heat.
3. Place chops on the grill, and cook for about 3 minutes per side until cooked through.
4. Serve warm.

Nutritional Facts: Calories 224, Fat 13g, Fiber 8.6g, Carbs 7g, Proteins 23g.

97. Rosemary cauliflower rolls

Prep time: 10 mins
Cooking time: 30 mins
Servings: 4
Ingredients:

- 1/3 cup of almond flour
- 4 cups of riced cauliflower
- 1/3 cup of reduced-fat, shredded mozzarella or cheddar cheese
- 2 eggs
- 2 Tbsp. of fresh rosemary, finely chopped
- ½ tsp. of salt

Directions:

1. Preheat your oven to 400 degrees F.
2. Combine all the listed ingredients in a medium-sized bowl.
3. Scoop the cauliflower mixture into 12 evenly-sized rolls/biscuits onto a lightly-greased and foil-lined baking sheet.
4. Bake until it turns golden brown, which should be achieved in about 30 minutes.
5. Note: if you want to have the outside of the rolls/biscuits crisp, then broil for some minutes before serving.

Nutritional Facts: Calories 254, Proteins 24g, Carbs 7g, Fat 8g.

98. Coconut chicken

Prep time: 10 mins
Cooking time: 5 mins
Servings: 4
Ingredients:

- 6 oz. chicken fillet
- ¼ cup of sparkling water
- 1 egg
- 3 Tbsp. coconut flakes
- 1 Tbsp. coconut oil
- 1 tsp. Greek seasoning

Directions:

1. Cut the chicken fillets into small pieces (nuggets).
2. Then crack the egg in the bowl and whisk it.
3. Mix up together the egg and sparkling water.
4. Add Greek seasoning and stir gently.
5. Dip the chicken nuggets in the egg mixture and then coat in the coconut flakes.
6. Melt the coconut oil in the skillet and heat it until it is simmering.
7. Then add the chicken nuggets.
8. Roast them for 1 minute from each side or until they are light brown.
9. Dry the cooked chicken nuggets with the help of a paper towel and transfer in the serving plates.

Nutritional Facts: Calories 141, Fat 8.9g, Fiber 0.3g, Carbs 1g, Proteins 13.9g.

CHAPTER 7:
Smoothies Recipes

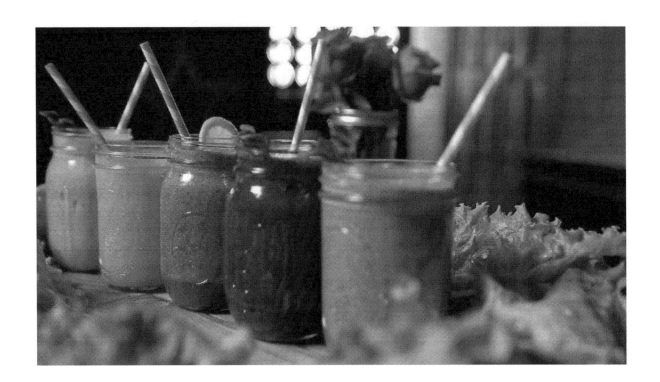

99. Beetroot & parsley smoothie

Prep time: 10 mins
Cooking time: 0 mins
Servings: 2
Ingredients:

- 1 cup carrot
- 1 cup beetroot
- 1 Tbsp. parsley
- 1 Tbsp. celery
- 1 cup ice

Directions:

1. In a blender. place all ingredients and blend until smooth.
2. Pour smoothie in a glass and serve.

Nutritional Facts: Calories 100, Fat 1g, Fiber 2g, Carbs 2g, Proteins 6g.

100. Coconut breezy shake dose

Prep time: 10 mins
Cooking time: 0 mins
Servings: 2
Ingredients:

- 1 cup skimmed milk (chilled)
- 1 cup pineapple chunks
- 4 Tbsp. shredded coconut
- Water as needed
- ½ scoop of vanilla protein powder

Directions:

1. Mix all the ingredients in a mixer and blend well for 20 seconds, until smooth texture is achieved.
2. Pour in a large glass and serve.

Nutritional Facts: Calories 476, Fat 40g, Fiber 9g, Carbs 33g, Proteins 6g.

101. Cashew boost smoothie

Prep time: 10 mins
Cooking time: 0 mins
Servings: 2
Ingredients:

- 2/4 cup raw cashews
- 1 cup chilled almond milk
- ¼ cup mixed fruit

Directions:

1. Blend together all ingredients and serve chilled.

Nutritional Facts: Calories 191, Fat 10g, Fiber 3g, Carbs 13g, Proteins 1g.

102.   Smooth root green cleansing smoothie

Prep time: 10 mins
Cooking time: 0 mins
Servings: 2
Ingredients:

- ½ cup fresh lettuce leaves
- ¼ green apple chunks
- A handful of cilantro
- ¼ lime juice
- Couple of cucumber slices
- 1 date without pit
- 1 cup chilled water

Directions:

1. Wash the apple and leaves well before use. Do not peel the apple; just remove the seeds and inedible parts.
2. Blend all the ingredients and serve.

Nutritional Facts: Calories 140, Fat 4g, Fiber 2g, Carbs 7g, Proteins 8g.

103. Twin berry smoothie

Prep time: 10 mins
Cooking time: 0 mins
Servings: 2
Ingredients:

- ½ cup peach chunks
- ¾ cup almond milk
- A handful of cranberries and raspberries
- Peel of an orange
- 1 scoop protein powder (whey)
- Ice cubes as required

Directions:

1. Chop the berries well, use natural orange peel, add all foods in a blender and blend well.
2. It's ready to serve.

Nutritional Facts: Calories 150, Fat 3g, Fiber 2g, Carbs 6g, Proteins 8g.

104. White bean smoothie to burn fats

Prep time: 10 mins
Cooking time: 0 mins
Servings: 2
Ingredients:

- 1 cup unsweetened rice milk (chilled)
- ¼ cup peach slices
- ¼ cup white beans cooked
- A pinch of cinnamon powder
- A pinch of nutmeg

Directions:

1. Pour milk in the blender and add the other ingredients.
2. Blend until smooth, then serve.

Nutritional Facts: Calories 150, Fat 3g, Fiber 2g, Carbs 6g, Proteins 8g.

105. Buttery banana shake

Prep time: 10 mins

Cooking time: 0 mins

Servings: 2

Ingredients:

- 1 Tbsp. raw peanut butter
- 1 cup almond milk
- 1 scoop protein powder any flavor
- ¼ cup Greek yogurt
- 1 tsp. basil
- 1 tsp. ginger paste
- 1 tsp. vanilla extract
- 1 tsp. sesame seeds

Directions:

1. Blend all ingredients in a blender.
2. Serve in the morning or evening after workouts.

Nutritional Facts: Calories 170, Fat 3g, Fiber 6g, Carbs 8g, Proteins 5g.

106. Grapefruit smoothie with cinnamon

Prep time: 10 mins

Cooking time: 0 mins

Servings: 2

Ingredients:

- 1 cup grapefruit juice, use pulp for fiber (optional)
- Ice cubes in crushed form as needed (2-3)
- 1 cinnamon stick
- 1 sliced banana
- 1 tsp. brown sugar

Directions:

1. Mix all ingredients in a blender and mix for 30 seconds to blend well.
2. Serve when done.

Nutritional Facts: Calories 170, Fat 3g, Fiber 6g, Carbs 8g, Proteins 5g.

107.   Carrot drink

Prep time: 10 mins
Cooking time: 0 mins
Servings: 2
Ingredients:

- 2 cups carrots
- 1 cup apple
- ½ tsp brown sugar

Directions:

1. In a blender, add all the ingredients and blend until smooth
2. Pour the smoothie in a glass and serve.

Nutritional Facts: Calories 140, Fat 4g, Fiber 2g, Carbs 7g, Proteins 8g.

108. Coconut cherry smoothie

Prep time: 10 mins
Cooking time: 0 mins
Servings: 2
Ingredients:

- 1 cup non-dairy coconut milk
- 4 ice cubes or as needed
- 1 cup mixed berries (blueberries, blackberries and cherries)
- ½ plantains
- A handful of mixed chopped fruits- pear/peach/guava
- 2 Tbsp. plain soy yogurt

Directions:

1. Toss in the berries, milk and other ingredients in a blender, and blend together well to make a smooth drink.
2. Serve in tall glasses.

Nutritional Facts: Calories 150, Fat 3g, Fiber 2g, Carbs 6g, Proteins 8g.

109.   Fats burning & water-based smoothie

Prep time: 10 mins
Cooking time: 0 mins
Servings: 2
Ingredients:

- 4 big strawberries
- 1 small piece of banana or an apple slice with peel
- ¼ tsp. of cinnamon powder
- 1 tsp. honey
- 2 cups water

Directions:

1. Take a blender and add water.
2. Remove stems from the berries and add in the blender.
3. Add cinnamon powder, honey, crushed ice cubes and the remaining fruit.
4. Blend and serve.

Nutritional Facts: Calories 170, Fat 3g, Fiber 6g, Carbs 8g, Proteins 5g.

110. Glory smoothie

Prep time: 10 mins
Cooking time: 0 mins
Servings: 2
Ingredients:

- ¼ cup kale
- A handful of romaine
- A handful of broccoli stems
- A celery stalk
- 1 cup juice of green apple
- 2 big cucumber slices
- ½ of a lemon juice and zest both

Directions:

1. This smoothie is Prepared by combining all ingredients listed above with juice and blending well.
2. Use ice or chilled juice to get a chilled drink.

Nutritional Facts: Calories 69, Fat 6.5g, Fiber 2.6g, Carbs 10.6g, Proteins 9.4g.

111. Grapes and peach smoothie

Prep time: 10 mins
Cooking time: 0 mins
Servings: 2
Ingredients:

- 1 cup red grapes juice
- 3 Tbsp. shredded coconut
- ½ scoop protein powder
- A handful of chopped pistachios
- 1 small guava and peach chopped
- Ice as required

Directions:

1. Mix all the ingredients in a blender and shake to make it a smooth drink.
2. Serve and enjoy the healthy treat.

Nutritional Facts: Calories 150, Fat 3g, Fiber 2g, Carbs 6g, Proteins 8g.

112.   Green tea purifying smoothie

Prep time: 10 mins
Cooking time: 0 mins
Servings: 2
Ingredients:

- 2 C. fresh baby spinach
- 3 C. frozen green grapes
- 1 medium ripe avocado peeled, pitted and chopped
- 2 tsp. organic honey
- 1½ C. strong brewed green tea

Directions:

1. In a high-speed blender, add all ingredients and pulse until smooth.
2. Transfer into serving glasses and serve immediately.

Nutritional Facts: Calories 476, Fat 40g, Fiber 9g, Carbs 33g, Proteins 6g.

113.   Kale batch detox smoothie

Prep time: 10 mins
Cooking time: 0 mins
Servings: 2
Ingredients:

- ¼ cup kale
- 1 cup chilled coconut water
- 2 pear slices
- ¼ cup avocado
- A handful of cilantro

Directions:

1. Blend all the ingredients in a blender for a minute and serve fresh.

Nutritional Facts: Calories 191, Fat 10g, Fiber 3g, Carbs 13g, Proteins 1g.

114. Lemon and garlic smoothie

Prep time: 10 mins
Cooking time: 0 mins
Servings: 2
Ingredients:

- 1 lemon juice
- 1 small clove of fresh garlic
- 1 glass water
- Few mint leaves
- 1 tsp. brown sugar

Directions:

1. Chop, slice or crush garlic clove and add in an electric mixer with water, lemon juice, sugar and mint leaves to blend and serve immediately.
2. It is better to serve this warm.

Nutritional Facts: Calories 170, Fat 3g, Fiber 6g, Carbs 8g, Proteins 5g.

115. Melon and nuts smoothie

Prep time: 10 mins
Cooking time: 0 mins
Servings: 2
Ingredients:

- 1 cup water melon chunks
- ¼ cup mixed nuts
- 1 cup soy milk
- ½ cup tofu
- Chilled water as needed
- 1 scoop of chocolate whey protein powder

Directions:

1. Blend all ingredients well to attain a smooth and soft drink.
2. Serve and enjoy.

Nutritional Facts: Calories 191, Fat 10g, Fiber 3g, Carbs 13g, Proteins 1g.

116. Muskmelon juice

Prep time: 10 mins
Cooking time: 0 mins
Servings: 2
Ingredients:

- 2 cups muskmelon
- 2 cups pineapple
- 1 cup ice

Directions:

1. In a blender, place all ingredients and blend until smooth.
2. Pour in a glass and serve.

Nutritional Facts: Calories 191, Fat 10g, Fiber 3g, Carbs 13g, Proteins 1g.

117. Oatmeal blast with fruit

Prep time: 10 mins
Cooking time: 0 mins
Servings: 2
Ingredients:

- ½ cup oats (steel cut)
- A pinch of ground cinnamon
- Ice cubes as needed
- 1 cup water
- ½ cup pineapple chunks

Directions:

1. Throw oats in a blender and slightly blend with water.
2. Add the fruit and other ingredients afterwards and blend again.

Nutritional Facts: Calories 150, Fat 3g, Fiber 2g, Carbs 6g, Proteins 8g.

118. Papaya juice

Prep time: 10 mins
Cooking time: 0 mins
Servings: 2
Ingredients:

- ½ cup papaya cubes
- ½ cup coconut
- ½ cup coconut water
- 1 cup ice

Directions:

1. In a blender, pour all the ingredients and blend until smooth
2. Pour the smoothie in a glass and serve.

Nutritional Facts: Calories 191, Fat 10g, Fiber 3g, Carbs 13g, Proteins 1g.

119.   Peach and kiwi smoothie

Prep time: 10 mins
Cooking time: 0 mins
Servings: 2
Ingredients:

- 1 cup plain low-fat yogurt
- ½ cup peach chunks
- 1 Tbsp. protein powder
- Water as needed
- ½ cup kiwi fruit

Directions:

1. Blend powder and fruits finely until you get a liquid consistency.
2. Serve chilled.

Nutritional Facts: Calories 151, Fat 7g, Fiber 12g, Carbs 9g, Proteins 20g.

120. Red capsicum juice

Prep time: 10 mins
Cooking time: 0 mins
Servings: 2
Ingredients:

- 1 cup red capsicum
- 1 cup carrot
- 1 cup apple
- 1 cup ice

Directions:

1. In a blender, add all the ingredients and blend until smooth
2. Pour the smoothie in a glass and serve.

Nutritional Facts: Calories 69, Fat 6.5g, Fiber 2.6g, Carbs 10.6g, Proteins 9.4g.

121.   Soothing smoothie for stomach

Prep time: 10 mins
Cooking time: 0 mins
Servings: 2
Ingredients:

- 1 tsp. brown sugar
- 1 tsp. lime juice
- 1 cup lite coconut milk
- ¾ cup papaya

Directions:

1. Pour the milk in an electric blender and mix in the lime juice, papaya and sugar.
2. Blend until smooth and serve. Add ice if you want it chilled.

Nutritional Facts: Calories 191, Fat 10g, Fiber 3g, Carbs 13g, Proteins 1g.

122. Triple C shake

Prep time: 10 mins
Cooking time: 0 mins
Servings: 2
Ingredients:

- ¼ cup raw spinach
- 1 Tbsp. cacao nibs
- 1 cup skimmed chocolate nut milk
- ¾ cup black or blue berries
- A dash of red pepper flakes
- A scoop of chocolate whey powder
- Water as needed
- 6 crushed ice cubes
- A handful of nuts
- A pinch of cinnamon powder

Directions:

1. Put all the ingredients in a blender and blend until smooth.
2. Serve chilled in a large glass and enjoy.

Nutritional Facts: Calories 476, Fat 40g, Fiber 9g, Carbs 33g, Proteins 6g.

CONCLUSION

Thank you for making it to the end! Due to the cirrhosis, your liver is unable to carry out one of its primary functions: ensuring that your body absorbs the nutrients it needs from the food you consume.

A cirrhosis diet can help you get the nutrients you need, ease the burden on your liver, ward off complications, and slow the progression of liver disease. Poor nutrition has been linked to an increased risk of cirrhosis-related consequences, including death, in persons with liver disease. Limiting liver disease's consequences and progression with a healthy diet and weight is possible. This diet also reduces the risk of diabetes and cardiovascular disease because of its ability to regulate blood sugar and lower blood pressure. When you eat healthily, your immune system is strengthened, which decreases your overall risk of being sick.

Keep in mind that liver illness is not terminal and can be controlled, so it's possible to still enjoy life. You should just take care of yourself by eating more naturally, limiting your sodium intake, and exercising for at least 30 minutes every day.

Have a wonderful day!

Made in the USA
Monee, IL
02 January 2023

24304015R00081